Psychiatric Emergencies
in Family Practice

Psychiatric Emergencies
in Family Practice

Edited by

John D Pollitt
MD FRCP FRCPsych DPM

Physician in Psychological Medicine and
Director of Medical Education
Hayes Grove Priory Hospital

Honorary Consulting Physician in Psychological Medicine
and formerly Physician in Charge
Department of Psychological Medicine
St Thomas' Hospital

formerly Assistant Director
British Postgraduate Medical Federation
(University of London)

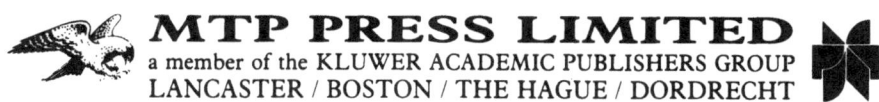
MTP PRESS LIMITED
a member of the KLUWER ACADEMIC PUBLISHERS GROUP
LANCASTER / BOSTON / THE HAGUE / DORDRECHT

Published in the UK and Europe by
MTP Press Limited
Falcon House
Lancaster, England

British Library Cataloguing-in-Publication Data

Psychiatric emergencies in family practice.
    1. Psychiatric emergencies   2. Family medicine
    I. Pollitt, John D.
    616.89'025   RC480.6

    ISBN-13: 978-94-010-7931-0

Published in the USA by
MTP Press
A division of Kluwer Academic Publishers
101 Philip Drive
Norwell, MA 02061, USA

Library of Congress Cataloging-in-Publication Data

Psychiatric emergencies in family practice.

    Includes bibliography and index.
    1. Psychiatric emergencies. 2. Family
medicine. I. Pollitt, John D. [DNLM: 1. Emergencies.
2. Family Practice. 3. Mental Health Services.
WM 401 P9736]
RC480.6.P7834   1987   616.89'025   87-2998
ISBN-13: 978-94-010-7931-0   e-ISBN-13: 978-94-009-3191-6
DOI: 10.1007/978-94-009-3191-6

Contents

List of Contributors

Dora Black, MD, FRCPsych, DPM
Consultant Child Psychiatrist, Royal Free Hospital, London
Honorary Consultant Psychiatrist, Hospital for Sick Children,
London

Ian F Brockington, MD, FRCPsych
Professor of Psychiatry, Head of Department of Psychiatry,
University of Birmingham

Kenneth Davison, FRCP, FRCP(Ed), FRCPsych, DPM
Consultant Psychiatrist, Newcastle General Hospital
Lecturer in Psychiatry, University of Newcastle

Robin Donald, MBChB, MRCGP, DPM, DObstRCOG
General Practitioner, formerly Associate Specialist in Psychiatry,
Tayside Area Alcoholism Unit, Sunnyside Road Hospital, Montrose,
Angus

Joan R Gomez, MB, FRCPsych, DPM
Consultant Psychiatrist, Westminster Hospital, London

Cyril Josephs, MD, FRCGP, DCH
General Practitioner,
Senior Medical Officer, Nightingale House, Clapham, London SW12

Maurice Lipsedge, MPhil, FRCP, FRCPsych
Consultant Psychiatrist, Guy's Hospital, London

John B Loudon, MBCHB, DPM, FRCPsych
Consultant Psychiatrist, Royal Edinburgh Hospital

Gillian C Mezey, MB, BS, MRCPsych
Senior Registrar in Psychiatry, The London and Maudsley Hospitals

Martin Mitcheson, MB, BCh, FRCPsych, DPM
Consultant Psychiatrist, Hereford Group of Hospitals

John Munro, MBChB, DObstRCOG, MRCGP
Medical Officer, University of Durham

Colin Murray Parkes, MD, FRCPsych
Consultant Psychiatrist, The London Hospital
Senior Lecturer, The London Hospital Medical School

John D Pollitt, MD, FRCP, FRCPsych, DPM
Consultant Physician in Psychological Medicine,
Hayes Grove Priory Hospital
Honorary Consulting Physician in Psychological Medicine,
St Thomas' Hospital, London

Alan Poole, BSc, MB, MRCP, FRCPsych, DPM
Consultant Psychiatrist, Tone Vale Hospital, Norton Fitzwarren,
Taunton, Somerset

Robert Romanis, MA, MB, BCh
General Practitioner, London

Kurt Schapira, MD, FRCP, FRCPsych, DPM
Consultant Psychiatrist, Royal Victoria Infirmary,
Newcastle-upon-Tyne
Lecturer, University of Newcastle-upon-Tyne
Sub-Dean, Royal College of Psychiatrists

Michael Swash, MD, FRCP, MRCPath
Consultant Neurologist, The London Hospital,
St Marks Hospital and Newham General Hospital, London

T G Tennent, DM, FRCPsych, DPM, Dip.Criminol.
14 Devonshire Place, London

Robina Thexton, MB, BS, MRCS, LRCP
Member of the Institute of Psychosexual Medicine,
Medical Officer for Ealing and Brent Youth Advisory Centres,
Psychosexual Counsellor at Margaret Pyke Centre, Soho Square,
London

Eric D West, FRCP, FRCPsych, DPM
Emeritus Consultant, Sutton Hospital, Surrey

David Will, BSc, MBChB, MRCPsych, Mem.SAAP
Consultant in Child and Adolescent Psychiatry,
Tayside Health Board
Honorary Senior Lecturer, Department of Psychiatry,
University of Dundee

Introduction

John D Pollitt

During the past 30 years, there has been a steady increase in the number of psychological and psychiatric problems identified and treated in general practice and referral to specialists has declined. Psychiatric emergencies are different, and even if the pace of life had not accelerated considerably, acute situations allow little time for reference. Some emergencies happen so infrequently that the average practitioner is unlikely to have a large fund of relevant past experience. Consequently, there is no opportunity for "battle drill".

This book is intended for the busy practitioner and it deals with urgent situations requiring a medical response. It is designed, for the most part, both for quick reference when appropriate and for more detailed consideration of the nature and background to many of the conditions leading to urgency. To facilitate locating the section concerned it is organised according to the presenting feature.

In dealing with urgent and difficult situations, recognition is perhaps of the greatest importance, and at the beginning of each chapter a local index, synopsis or quick reference page is provided to enable doctors to refer rapidly to problems presented over the telephone or directly in the surgery or patient's home. The chapters themselves provide a framework in which to set each urgent situation so that the doctor can be in a better position to understand what is likely to happen, rather than simply transfer the patient to a specialist, hospital or paramedical agency as a routine. In many chapters sufficient information is given to enable the family practitioner to manage situations personally. In others, when the patient should be referred or placed under section, precise instructions are given for management.

The authors include both general practitioners or those practising in a similar context and specialists in certain fields. All have been chosen because of their particular interest. No attempt has been made to produce a stereotyped format, or to promote equal emphasis in all sections. There is a degree of overlap, which has been retained on the basis that for emergencies "what is worth saying is worth repeating". In other places different authors deal with the same problem in different ways. Psychiatry is still properly viewed from many angles, and just as elective situations can be resolved by many different approaches, psychiatric emergencies, as described here, demonstrate a number of different viewpoints, many different styles and many ways of communicating doctor to doctor. Not only does this emphasise the breadth of the subject, but it also conveys a subtlety of feeling which is very close to matters of motivation which guide us all in a lifetime of practice.

It is hoped that not only family practitioners, but also senior and junior psychiatric staff will find matters of interest here. In some cases there have been considerable advances during the past few years and these chapters will be found helpful in the sense of up-dating.

Having practised psychiatry for 35 years I found, in every contribution by others, a richness of new information, ideas, fresh approaches and facts, and it is hoped that this will refresh the busy practitioner, provide him or her with a guide to emergencies which will increase confidence in managing situations of the type in which only the cognoscent can shine, and add to the purely professional sense of reward.

It remains for me to thank all the contributors for their efforts and artistry and for the enjoyment of reading their work, and to express gratitude to the publishers, and to my secretary Pauline Trinder, for their accommodating flexibility, tolerance and thoughtfulness throughout.

1

Deluded patients

Kurt Schapira

QUICK REFERENCE GUIDE

THE IMPORTANCE OF AN ADJECTIVE

Psychiatric terms readily find their way into everyday vocabulary and en passage lose their specific meaning. Thus, "delusions" became other people's beliefs with which we strongly disagree or of which we disapprove. Not so in clinical practice; to describe some one as being deluded has important implications because it denotes the presence of a **serious mental illness** and one that often brings with it **special problems in management**.

WHAT IS A DELUSION?

A number of features characterise a delusion:

1. It is a **false belief**. Exceptionally, the patient's belief may be correct but the evidence upon which it is based is both unreasonable and irrational. The truth of the belief is seen by the patient as self-evident and requiring no proof.
2. It is held with **absolute conviction** which resists change or modification, despite evidence to the contrary.
3. It is **not in keeping with the person's intellectual, social and cultural background**, nor is it shared by members of his ethnic, religious or cultural group.
4. The theme of the delusion is **often fantastic** or at least, highly unlikely.
5. Often the delusion has **great personal significance** for the patient.

Delusions arise from morbid internal mental processes, the nature of which is as yet little understood. Hence their failure to be modified either by argument or by experience.

Finally, the way in which a false belief emerges and the nature of the reasons that are given for its acceptance are as important characteristics of its delusional nature as any of the other features.

BELIEFS THAT ARE NOT DELUSIONAL

Strong beliefs which to others are patently false are held by all of us. They may concern any aspect of life and often are beliefs shared with members of our cultural, social, ethnic, political or religious group. One of their main characteristics is that they are often not amenable to change by the most reasonable of arguments or evidence.

Delusions **must** also **be distinguished from over-valued ideas**. These are deeply held convictions not shared by others which can, however, be understood in terms of the background of an individual and his past experience. Many ideas about the causes of some illnesses and their treatment with a variety of totally untested remedies, belong to the category of over-valued ideas. Often, the more irrational such beliefs are, the more firmly they are held. Although the distinction between a true delusion and an over-valued idea may not always be easy to make, in practice this should not present any real difficulties since delusions are only one symptom of a psychotic illness; other symptoms will help resolve any diagnostic problem.

WHAT KIND OF DELUSION?

Delusions may arise de novo - the patient experiences a sudden realisation, the nature of which is inexplicable in terms of anything that is happening in his environment. The idea appears like an instant brainwave, an absolute and unshakeable new piece of knowledge and "understanding". Such delusions are termed **primary** or **autochthonous** - they spring, as did Minerva, fully-formed from the head of Jupiter.

An example of a primary delusion was expressed by a bus driver who, on finding that the third set of traffic lights he was approaching that morning had turned red, took this to signify that he had been canonized. Nothing apart from the morbid mental process of the patient could possibly bridge the gap between these two events. To the patient, the truth of his belief was self-evident.

In contrast, **secondary delusions** can be understood as deriving from a previous morbid experience. Thus, secondary delusions usually follow a primary delusion, so that the bus driver, having been canonized, now acknowledges the smiles of his passengers and the signals of the policeman on traffic control duty, as approriate signs of homage.

Secondary delusions may also arise on the basis of a morbid mood change. Thus, a profoundly depressed patient with marked feelings of guilt may be convinced that the ambulance, which he was told would take him to hospital, will in fact take him to prison.

On the other hand, a morbidly elated and joyful mood is likely to be accompanied by grandiose delusions, when the patient believes himself to be endowed with superhuman powers or abilities, or to be a personage of great renown.

As the number of secondary delusions increases, a delusional system may emerge in which each delusional idea can be understood in the light of the preceding one.

THE THEME OR CONTENT OF DELUSIONS

It is helpful in clinical practice to classify delusions according to their themes, since these provide a pointer, but nothing more, to the diagnosis of the underlying mental illness.

Persecutory (often called paranoid) delusions
(see also pp.14,15,16)

These occur most commonly in schizophrenia but can be a symptom of the affective psychosis and of organic states, delirium or dementia. Paranoid delusions may also occur in alcohol or drug-induced paranoid states. Persecutory delusions most commonly implicate individuals or organisations held by the patient to be intent on inflicting harm or spreading malicious lies about him. The resentment and anger with which the schizophrenic patient responds to these activities may lead him to complain to the authorities or attack those he believes to be involved.

The psychologically depressed patient, on the other hand, often readily accepts this "persecution" which he regards as a just retribution for past misdemeanors (usually fictitious), which he believes have become known to everyone around him (see also Chapter 5).

In acute organic states, delirium, persecutory delusions frequently occur but the theme of these, as in dementia, is often determined by the premorbid personality of the patient. Delusions tend to be transient and often poorly defined; they mirror the fluctuating state of consciousness.

Delusions concerning the possession of thought

These are of three kinds and are **pathognomonic of schizophrenia:**

(a) Thought Insertion

The patient believes that his thoughts are not the product of his own mind and that they have been implanted by some outside agency.

(b) Thought Withdrawal

Here the patient believes that his thoughts have been taken out of his mind. This belief may be seen as representing an explanation for the process of thought-blocking, in which the flow of thought of the patient is interrupted.

(c) Thought Broadcasting

The patient believes that other people are aware of his thoughts and have received this information via the television, radio, or occasionally some other magical process, such as thought transference (see also p.16).

Delusions of reference

Patients with this kind of delusion believe that events or the behaviour of other people have a **special personal significance.** Often they are identified as broadcasting to the world some derogatory aspect (true or fictitious) of the patient's past. Thus a television play on the subject of homosexuality is seen by the patient as intending, and indeed, succeeding in letting everyone know that he is a homosexual.

Delusions of jealousy (also called "Othello syndrome")

This syndrome is more common among men. It bespeaks not a mere jealous or suspicious nature but a delusional belief that misconduct is taking place, often with the most unlikely persons. Evidence is continually sought by the patient to support his allegations. Violent

4

behaviour often ensues and may be provoked by the false confession of the spouse made in the vain hope of peace from constant interrogation. The promise of forgiveness is a snare; such confessions may result in homicide.

Delusions of guilt and unworthiness

Often called Depressive Delusions - they are the hallmark of severe depressive illness. The patient is convinced that because of a minor misdemeanor (real or imagined) retribution in the form of public disgrace, prison or even death will be visited upon him or his family. Such delusions often lead to **suicide** and even to homicide, as in cases of infanticide occurring in the setting of a post-natal depressive psychosis.

Nihilistic delusions

These represent extreme feelings of pessimism and hopelessness about the present and future. Often these ideas relate to past events, retrospective falsification, such as the patient who obtained a First Class Honours Degree some years previously, and who came to believe that this was due to the fact that he erroneously received the marks of another candidate. Nihilistic delusions may also take a somatic form, when the patient believes that his bowels or circulation have ceased to work.

Hypochondriacal delusions

These represent an **unshakeable belief of illness,** contrary to all medical evidence, often supported by an exhaustive number of investigations. Such beliefs may be life-long and often originate with a history of being "frail and delicate" in childhood and receiving much solicitous care from parents and doctors.

When occurring for the first time in adult and late life, such delusions are often the most prominent symptoms of a depressive illness; they commonly comprise preoccupations with cancer or other diseases regarded by the patient as incurable and hopeless. Viral Hepatitis and in more recent years AIDS have been added to the repertoire of hypochondriacal preoccupations, often such ideas are linked with much self blame relating to the patient's own lack of initiative which might have prevented such catastrophies. Depressed patients with hypochondriacal delusions have a particularly high risk of committing suicide (see also p.54).

Delusions of poverty

Once quite common are now seen only rarely, occurring mainly among the elderly where they account for some of the cases of self-denial and gross self neglect inspite of more than adequate, and at times considerable financial means. It is an erroneous belief that this condition occurs exclusively among the traditionally par-simonious Scots!

Grandiose delusions

Like depressive delusions these are congruous with the prevailing mood. The patient believes himself to be a personage of renown, great wealth or unique and unusual abilities. These ideas may be combined as in the case of a patient who claimed he had, following the recognition that he was a genius, received 10 million pounds for a brilliant plan he had conceived for reorganising the Health Service! Such delusions may be expressed in a light-hearted vein but nevertheless represent deeply held and unshakeable convictions as evidenced by the irritability and anger which meets any expression of doubt as to their veracity.

Strange religious ideas in members of small minority religious and cults, although uncommonly met with in clinical practice, deserve special mention. Consultation with another member of the group is advisable before deciding whether the belief represents a delusion in the clinical sense (see above).

DIAGNOSIS

The presence of a delusion denotes **a psychotic illness**. Indeed the patient may suffer from any of the three major psychoses: **schizophrenia, manic-depressive psychosis**, or **organic psychosis**. Apart from the theme of the delusion which may give a pointer to the diagnosis, independent features upon which the diagnosis is made must be present. Table 1 illustrates the relationship between the theme (or content) of the delusion and the clinical diagnosis, and underlines the considerable diagnostic overlap.

A comprehensive account of the psychoses is not possible in the context of this chapter; the following will serve as a useful guide:

Is consciousness clouded? If there is evidence of "clouding" i.e. there is disorientation in time and place, often episodic, then a diagnosis of delirium, an acute organic state, should be made and the underlying organic pathology be sought (see also chapter 20).

In dementia, symptoms of intellectual and memory deterioration accompanied by a decline in social functioning are usually to be found. Occasionally, however, paranoid delusions may be the presenting symptom of a dementing process.

Table 1   DIAGNOSIS AND THEME OF DELUSION

THEME OF DELUSION	SCHIZOPHRENIA	AFFECTIVE PSYCHOSES		ORGANIC PSYCHOSES	
		Depression	Mania	Delirium	Dementia
Persecutory delusion (Paranoid)	+	±	±	+	+
Delusions concerning possession of thought	+	-	-	-	-
Delusions of reference	+	±	±	±	±
Delusions of jealousy (Othello syndrome)	±	-	-	-	±
Delusions of guilt and worthlessness	-	+	-	-	±
Grandiose delusions	±	-	+	±	±
Hypochondriacal delusions	±	+	±	-	+

In a clear sensorium, i.e. in the absence of clouding of consciousness, the differential diagnosis lies between schizophrenia and affective psychosis. Apart from other clinical features in support of either diagnosis, the content, i.e. the theme of the delusion, with the noteable exception of those concerned with possession of thought which are pathognomonic of schizophrenia, is of relatively little value in distinguishing between the two conditions.

MANAGEMENT

First steps

It is often the very nature of delusions that will prevent the patient from seeking help; he does not perceive them as different from his other beliefs. Only when unpleasant in nature, as with persecutory or depressive delusions, do they become the subject of complaint. In most cases, however, it will be others who will ask for help because of the bizarre or dangerous behaviour of the patient.

Patients who have had previous psychotic illness are aware that their beliefs are considered abnormal and may become quite skilful in hiding them. However, their behaviour and often indirect evidence from what they say, clearly indicates that the delusions have returned or are still persisting.

The interview

When false beliefs emerge in the course of the history it is important to ascertain how profoundly they are held. It is the unshakeable quality of the belief which constitutes one of the important

7

characteristics of a delusion; there is no "as if" quality to it.

The initial interview requires a great deal of patience and tact on the part of the doctor if confidence is to be established and the patient helped. It is a vital step in the subsequent management. The patient who may well be suspicious and distrustful should be allowed to speak freely and the doctor must register neither surprise nor incredulity at some of the things that he hears. **Delusional ideas should neither be contradicted, argued about, nor indeed agreed with by the doctor,** inspite of occasional pressure from the patient to do so. Often changing the subject of the conversation will delay confrontation and so avoid abrupt termination of the interview by the patient. If all fails, an "agree to differ" arrangement combined with a rapid change to another topic is often the best policy.

Delusions relating to thought processes and to volition and control are sometimes difficult to elicit and questions must be carefully phrased. Thus, if one wishes to ascertain whether the patient is experiencing "thought insertion" an appropriate question would be: "Have you ever felt some of the thoughts in your mind were not your own but were put there from outside?" The patient's answer should then be recorded verbatim. The recording of symptoms, particularly of psychotic symptoms, in the patient's own words is a vital part of history taking because it has diagnostic significance.

The recording of symptoms in the patient's own words, particularly when these are psychotic symptoms, is far more helpful than a statement to the effect that the patient was deluded.

Similarly, if a patient produces a positive response to any question relating to a psychotic symptom, it is important to encourage him to elaborate. Only then may a network of a delusional system be revealed.

At the end of the clinical interview the following questions should be answered:

1. Is the patient deluded?
2. What is the clinical diagnosis?
3. What are the other clinical features in support of the diagnosis?
4. Will the patient accept treatment voluntarily?
5. If not, is he likely to act on his delusions and would he then be a danger to himself or to others?

The answer to the last question will determine whether the patient must be admitted to hospital.

ADMISSION TO HOSPITAL

On a voluntary basis

If the patient can be persuaded to come into hospital this course should always be taken:

1. It permits a full diagnostic assessment, particularly where a possibility of an organic psychosis arises.
2. Effective treatment can be achieved more speedily.
3. It relieves the family of much anxiety.
4. There must always be some degree of uncertainty as to when a delusional belief may precipitate antisocial or aggressive behaviour.

The consequences of the socially disruptive behaviour of psychotic patients can be considerable, and often have to be faced by the patient once he has recovered.

Compulsory admission

If the answer to question 5 is in the affirmative and he refuses admission, compulsory admission under **Section 2** of the Mental Health Act (Application for Assessment - 28 days) is indicated. This procedure requires:

i. Application by the **patient's nearest relative** or an approved Social Worker who must have seen the patient within the last 14 days.
ii. A medical recommendation by **two doctors,** one of whom must be approved under Section 12 of the Mental Health Act.

In emergencies, a simpler procedure **Section 4** (Emergency Order for Assessment - 72 hours) of the Mental Health Act should be invoked. This only requires:

i. Application by the nearest relative **or** approved Social Worker.
ii. Medical recommendation by **one doctor** who must have seen the patient within the previous 24 hours. This doctor need not be approved under Section 12 of the Act.

The presence of a delusion as part of a psychiatric illness confers **special problems** as regards effective management. **Patience, tact, and skill** in the initial interview is vital as is the need to **act promptly** in collaboration with other professional colleagues.

EXAMPLES

Delusions of jealousy	"My wife has been with every man in our street this past week".
Grandiose delusions	"I have the wisdom of Solomon and the strength of Goliath". (a frail and dementing octagenarian)
Hypochondriacal delusions	"I am riddled with a cancer which all the Specialists I have seen have failed to find".

(continued)

9

Possession of thought	"There is a gadget inside the Television in the ward which reads my thoughts day and night".
Delusions of persecution	"When I leave the house I am followed by two men in a black car wearing hats. One is a KGB man and the other an American Secret Agent".
Delusions of reference	"The Radio Series "World Power" has been especially produced to let every one know that I have lost my sexual powers".
Delusions of guilt, ruin and poverty	"I can never be forgiven for what I have done. I am bankrupt and my family will starve. I am beyond the human pale and deserve to be punished". (when objective testimony shows the patient to be a successful, comfortably off business man, devoted to his family.)

2

Suspicious patients

Kenneth Davison

QUICK REFERENCE GUIDE

THE SORTING PROCESS

Is the suspiciousness lifelong or recent?

A. Lifelong suspiciousness
   This usually indicates a paranoid personality.

   i. Is the patient's attitude and behaviour par for the course?
       = another manifestation of **personality reaction**. Remember that the patient's grievances may sometimes be genuine.

11

    ii. Is the patient's reaction more intense than usual or are the ideas expressed delusional? Consider: **paranoid reaction, paranoid psychosis, depressive illness** or **occult physical illness**.

B. Recent suspiciousness

    i. **Young adult**
        a.   Is the suspiciousness episodic and variable? Consider: **drug abuse** with **glue sniffing, LSD, cocaine, cannabis** or **amphetamines**.
        b.   Is there eccentricity, social withdrawal, bizarre delusions, auditory hallucinations, incoherent thought, fatuous giggling and feelings of outside control? Consider: **schizophrenia**.

    ii. **Age 30 to 60 years**
        a.   Does the patient hold bizarre beliefs without hallucinations but appear otherwise a normal person? Consider: **paranoia**.
        b.   Does the patient express persecutory delusions and experience auditory hallucinations? Consider: **paranoid schizophrenia, alcohol abuse, paranoid reaction to prescribed drugs, epileptic psychosis**.
        c.   Has the suspiciousness developed very suddenly in association with fluctuating awareness, disorientation in time and/or place, noisy restless nights and possibly visual hallucinations? Consider: **delirium** due to **physical illness, alcohol or sedative withdrawal** or **confusional reaction to prescribed drugs**.
        d.   Is there evidence of preceding gradual decline in efficiency, memory impairment or disinhibited behaviour? Consider: **pre-senile dementia, cerebral tumour, hypothyroidism, or primary mood disorder**.

    iii. **Elderly person (>60 years)**
        a.   Is the person deaf or living alone? Consider: **paraphrenia**.
        b.   Is there associated forgetfulness, declining self-care and intellectual impairment? Consider: **senile or vascular dementia**.
        c.   Has there been a sudden deterioration in coping ability with muddled thinking, disorientation in time and place, restless nights, and possibly visual hallucinations? Consider: **drug intoxication, delirium due to physical disease**.
        d.   Is there associated depression with ideas of guilt and worthlessness and disturbance of appetite and sleep? Consider: **depressive illness**.

INTERVIEWING THE SUSPICIOUS PATIENT

Suspiciousness is, fortunately, not a common feature of the medical consultation for when it occurs it is seriously disruptive of the doctor-patient relationship which is normally based on mutual trust. It is an important attitude to detect as it may be not only a personality trait but also an early symptom of serious mental or physical illness.

Suspiciousness may be all-pervasive and directed at everyone in the immediate environment, including the doctor. In other cases suspicion is more selectively aroused by specific individuals or groups, commonly the spouse, neighbours, workmates, employer, the Police, etc. when the attitude to the doctor is often one of conspiratorial confiding and the patient is only too ready to tell his story. Difficulties arise when suspicion is directed at the doctor, either as an individual, a representative of his profession or as part of a general suspiciousness of everyone.

The **first encounter** with a suspicious patient is **crucial** and may determine whether he will accept help or treatment. The patient's initial reaction may vary from sullen, obdurate silence to a stream of hostile abuse. His prevailing mood is usually one of anxiety, tension and hypersensitivity with a tendency to find sinister motives or critical meaning in the most innocent remarks or actions. The patient should be put at ease and reassured as far as possible but remember that humorous or facetious comments are not well received. The possibility of personal violence should not be ignored.

It is wise not to take notes during the interview as this often arouses suspicion and leads to a demand to read them. Information from a relative or friend is necessary to complete the picture but should be obtained separately as the patient rarely allows anyone else to be interviewed out of his presence.

SPECIAL PROBLEMS WITH SUSPICIOUS PATIENTS

1. Refusal to accept hospital admission
    In the last resort compulsory admission under the Mental Health Act may be necessary but patients can sometimes be persuaded to enter hospital informally if the invitation is couched in non-threatening terms. "You need a break from all this hassle", or "I can see your nerves have been badly upset by these events" are often surprisingly effective lines to take.
2. Refusal to accept medication
    The patient is often reluctant to accept medication either because of a fear of being poisoned or because he does not accept that he is ill. The comment about the patient's nerves mentioned in item 1 may succeed, otherwise reference to the patient's over-sensitive mind and the need to insulate it against external assaults is a useful ploy.
3. Refusal to allow access to the patient's home
    Some patients are so suspicious that they refuse to allow anyone

13

into the house. If a relative or friend is unable to persuade them to undo the barricades the local Social Services Department should be informed as Section 135 of the Mental Health Act, which allows forcible access by a constable on a magistrate's warrant to premises where a person believed to be suffering from mental disorder, being unable to care for himself, is living alone, may need to be invoked.

WHAT MAKES PATIENTS SUSPICIOUS?

Suspiciousness is a feature of the paranoid state of which there are several types.

The paranoid personality

Personality represents the sum of the motivational and temperamental qualities of an individual leading to a characteristic mode of perceiving and reacting to the environment. The paranoid personality habitually reacts by employing the mental mechanism of projection resulting in the attribution to others of the individual's own thoughts and feelings. He over-reacts to the daily experiences of life with a sense of humiliation for which he blames the machinations of others. General mistrust and readiness to take offence lead to social isolation. Mild disagreements are perceived as rejection and alleged injustices are catalogued and long remembered leading to a persistently resentful attitude. He is never happier than when engaged in a struggle, usually to prove himself right and someone else wrong, not infrequently the doctor. The patient questions every medical decision and will insist on endless further opinions. He is a great complainer and letters to the FPC, GMC, BMA, MP, PM or even the Queen are distinctive elements in his repertoire.
    The doctor's reaction is often one of anger as he feels his competence is being repeatedly questioned. Equanimity is best retained by accepting the mistrust, suspicion, subtle insults and accusations as an intractable modus operandi that the patient is powerless to change.

The paranoid reaction

The paranoid reaction is an exaggerated response to disappointing or humiliating circumstances displayed by certain sensitive individuals, such as those with paranoid personalities, and by some normal personalities in special circumstances. Brief feelings of being the centre of attention or being looked at or talked about when entering a pub or restaurant are quite common. These feelings only become morbid when they persist, carry conviction and become elaborated in delusional fashion.

14

The paranoid reaction is really a transient psychosis that is differentiated from the paranoid sub-groups of schizophrenia by its intelligibility in the light of the circumstances and personality of the subject.

A paranoid reaction is the likely diagnosis when the premorbid personality is known to have been of paranoid type or where there is a special disability such as physical disfigurement or sexual deviation or special circumstances such as membership of a religious or ethnic minority. The prognosis for these reactions is good as they usually respond to removal of the precipitating stress although the patient remains vulnerable to future recurrence.

Paranoid psychoses

These are specific illnesses distinguished by the occurrence of **delusions** and sometimes **auditory hallucinations,** and the absence of significant mood change or intellectual impairment. Delusions are false unshakeable beliefs out of keeping with a person's social and cultural background.

The finer points of psychiatric differential diagnosis are of rather academic importance as treatment is basically the same, viz. a neuroleptic drug. Nevertheless the following syndromes are recognized:

Paranoia

This is characterized by a **fixed belief** or **set of beliefs** of a **persecutory or grandiose nature** without the development of hallucinations. Specific examples are:

1. Litigious paranoia
   This merges imperceptibly with the paranoid personality group and is only distinguished by a greater departure from reality and grosser and more bizarre misrepresentation of events. These patients don't know when to stop and will take apparently minor grievances to ever higher authorities. Many pursue redress in the Courts often at considerable financial sacrifice. Alleged medical mismanagement often figures in their paranoid fantasies and the doctor should therefore refrain from any comment that might be interpreted as critical of other doctors or their past management of the patient.

2. Paranoid jealousy (Othello syndrome)
   Again this overlaps with personality disorder as many insecure men are extremely possessive of their wives or girl-friends and become very angry if they look at or talk to another man, no matter how innocently.
   The psychotically jealous man develops the conviction that his wife is unfaithful and bolsters his belief with all manner of flimsy evidence. (Occasionally the roles are reversed and the

wife is morbidly jealous of her husband.) Thus he times her when she goes shopping, follows her to work and searches for seminal stains on her underwear or the bedclothes. Attempts to extort a confession from the unfortunate spouse are made, often with the employment of violence. Homicide is an ever-present risk, hence this condition should never be taken lightly. Specialist advice should be obtained.

Although often arising de novo, paranoid jealousy can also be associated with depressive illness and/or alcohol abuse.

Paranoid schizophrenia(see also p.52)

This is a form of schizophrenia with onset over age 30 years, characterized by prominent **persecutory delusions** and **auditory hallucinations** but with little, if any personality deterioration or disruption of thought processes. Like other forms of schizophrenia there is no clouding of consciousness or impairment of memory or intellect. Ideas of persecution by neighbours, workmates, or some agency such as the Police, Communists or Freemasons are common. The patient has the feeling of being the centre of attention and the most banal events appear to be directed at him. He finds himself referred to on radio and TV and the lyrics of pop songs carry a hidden message. Voices are heard talking amongst themselves about the patient and making critical remarks or commenting on his actions.

Some younger schizophrenics appear suspicious and perplexed but they are recognized by their eccentricity, social withdrawal, bizarre delusions and auditory hallucinations, incoherent thought processes, fatuous giggling and feelings of outside control.

Delusional misidentification is a specific symptom manifested as the belief that close relatives and friends, and sometimes the doctor, are all impostors (the Capgras syndrome) or that a particular individual is masquerading in a variety of disguises (the Frégoli syndrome). These syndromes can also be associated with organic brain disease.

Paraphrenia (late paraphrenia, persistent persecutory state of the elderly)

This term is applied to a paranoid psychosis without depressive or organic features developing after 60 years in well-preserved personalities. An association with deafness and social isolation has been identified.

The elderly person becomes convinced that her neighbours or relatives are interfering with her and attempting to harm her or drive her out of her home. Neighbours are overheard uttering threats or commenting adversely on the patient's character and behaviour. Complaints of nocturnal visitations for criminal or sexual purposes are common and more bizarre allegations, such as the release of poisonous gas under the floorboards, may develop.

The patient's initial response is usually to call the Police or demand to be re-housed and it is usually a worried relative who calls the doctor. A common problem is then the refusal of the patient to let anyone into the house (see above).

Intoxications

Intoxication due to drugs or alcohol may evoke suspiciousness by either inducing a delirious (confusional) state or a paranoid psychosis of the type already described. An **intoxication** should be considered **when suspiciousness develops suddenly in a previously normal person**.

In a young person consider drug abuse involving glue or solvent sniffing, cannabis, LSD, "magic mushrooms" (containing the hallucinogen psilocybin), cocaine or amphetamines. In older patients prescribed drugs or alcohol are more likely causes.

Drug-induced delirium (toxic confusional state, acute organic psychosis, acute brain syndrome)

This is particularly common in the elderly and concurrent physical disease may add to the problem. There is clouding of consciousness manifested as disorientation in time and/or place, noisy restlessness at night, irritability, a suspicious, hostile attitude and sometimes visual hallucinations. Ill-defined fleeting persecutory delusions are common and there may be accompanying incontinence, ataxia and falling attacks.

Almost any drug can produce this effect but the commonest are sedatives, hypnotics, major tranquillisers, diuretics, digoxin and anti-Parkinson agents. Drugs of abuse can also be implicated as can sudden withdrawal of a habitually taken drug, especially barbiturates, benzodiazepines, chlormethiazole ("Heminevrin") and alcohol (see also chapter 20).

Drug-induced paranoid psychoses (toxic psychoses)

These resemble the spontaneously-occurring paranoid psychoses previously described. In contrast to delirium there is no clouding of conciousness and the age distribution is more widely dispersed.

Again almost any drug can be implicated but the prescribed drugs commonly involved are steroids, L-dopa, bromocriptine, indomethacin and appetite supressant drugs. Alcohol or amphetamine abuse are potent causes of paranoid psychosis.

OTHER CAUSES OF SUSPICIOUSNESS

Primary mood disorder

Some patients with severe depressive illness also develop paranoid ideas such as believing they are being spied upon and talked about. Typical depressive symptoms will be in evidence.

17

Suspiciousness may be an early sign of the development of puer-peral psychosis, most likely in the first 2 weeks after childbirth. This is often a mixture of depressive and paranoid symptoms and is important because of the risk of suicide and infanticide.

Some manic patients can also be inordinately suspicious but will be recognized by their elevated mood, increased activity, rapid speech and general air of bombastic grandiosity.

Physical illness

The physical illnesses most often associated with pure paranoid states are endocrine disorders such as hypo- and hyper-thyroidism and Cushing's syndrome. Other physical illnesses can induce paranoia as a symptom of delirium as described above. These are commoner in the elderly and include infections and cardiac, renal or hepatic failure.

Organic brain disease

Suspiciousness is a common early feature of organic brain disease. The forgetful patient easily develops the idea that someone is deliberately hiding or stealing her possessions. In the elderly this is usually due to senile or vascular dementia. In younger patients pre-senile dementia due to conditions such as Alzheimer's disease and Huntington's chorea or primary or secondary brain tumours are possibilities.

A paranoid psychosis is associated with temporal lobe epilepsy and a transient paranoid state can occur after an epileptic fit.

Suspicious patients, therefore, deserve to be taken seriously and not ignored, as a suspicious attitude may conceal a wide spectrum of mental and physical pathology.

3

Alcoholic patients

Robin Donald

QUICK REFERENCE GUIDE

ACUTE PROBLEMS PRESENTED BY ALCOHOLIC PATIENTS IN FAMILY PRACTICE

1. **Acute intoxication**
   A drunk patient may be argumentative and abusive. Never try and reason with a patient in this state - it is not worth it! If a patient is violent or threatening violence, have no hesitation in calling the police if anyone is in real danger of assault. A person who is stuporose or comatose as a result of alcohol intoxication should be placed in the "recovery position", because of the risk of inhaling vomit.

2. **Alcohol withdrawal state**
   In general practice alcoholic emergencies are generally associated with an alcohol withdrawal state, e.g.

   a. Withdrawal fits - remember the possibility of alcohol abuse if a middle-aged patient has an unexplained major convulsion.

b. Delirium tremens - a typical patient exhibiting this is a heavy-smoking publican with a chest infection.
c. Wernicke's encephalopathy - an elderly confused patient with an intercurrent illness may have been drinking excessively and neglecting his nutrition.
d. Parasuicide and suicide are often associated with alcohol problems.

Alcohol is now the great mimic in medicine, and it is no respecter of age, sex, social class or occupation. The doctor must always be on his guard for its far-reaching effects. **Never try and treat medically a patient with an alcohol problem while that patient is still drinking.**

ALCOHOLISM AND MENTAL DISORDER

Amnesias ("blackouts") - frequently experienced by people with serious drinking problems; but also by social drinkers who have drunk unwisely on occasions.

Withdrawal fits - Grand Mal convulsions associated with sudden reduction of alcohol consumption, often several fits within 2-3 days; may be followed by Delirium tremens.

Alcoholic hallucinosis -
a. Fleeting, transient hallucinations - auditory or visual: associated with continued drinking and also withdrawal of alcohol.
b. Persistent and repetitive auditory hallucinations without delirium, associated with continued drinking. The hallucinations may however persist for some months after patient becomes abstinent before gradually fading. Condition not always manifest without specific and careful questioning.

Delirium tremens ("shakes" and "horrors")

Features   -   Delirium
            -    Tremor, which may affect whole body
            -    Marked restlessness, with pressure of activity
            -    Visual hallucinations: frequently rats and snakes; often Lilliputian figures seen on bed; patterns on wallpaper and carpets may assume grotesque shapes
            -    Alternating terror and cheerfulness
            -    Vestibular disturbances
            -    Profuse sweating which may lead to dehydration

Delirium tremens is often associated with physical illness e.g. infection, or sudden withdrawal of alcohol after trauma or surgery. On recovery the patient may have a clear recollection of his symptoms.

Morbid jealousy - most often sexual jealousy, delusions of spouse's infidelity - the Othello syndrome, which can lead to senseless acts of violence (see also p.15).

Wernicke-Korsakov syndrome:
Wernicke's encephalopathy - the classical triad of clouding of consciousness, ataxia and ophthalmoplegia not always seen: due to thiamine deficiency, the condition will readily respond to parenteral doses of thiamine and other vitamins of B complex (i.v. Parentrovite).
Korsakov's psychosis - may develop insidiously, or follow Delirium tremens or Wernicke syndrome.
Characteristics   - Grossly impaired memory for recent events
                   - Increase in emotional lability
                   - Confabulation - false accounting for activities
Treat with parenteral thiamine, 50 mg daily for several weeks, then weekly for 6 months. Prognosis variable.

Alcoholic dementia - nowadays recognized as an insidious and non-specific type of alcohol-related brain damage. Initially may present with some mild memory defect and impairment of judgment; without treatment may proceed to full-blown dementia with irreversible brain damage.

Depression - feelings of depression may be caused by excessive drinking; and a depressive illness may cause alcohol abuse. It is important to clarify the situation and make a definite diagnosis, especially as there may be a risk of SUICIDE. The clinical picture should become clear when the patient abstains from alcohol and anti-depressant medication should never be offered while the patient is still drinking.

Phobic anxiety states - acute anxiety in certain situations. Alcohol often used in self-medication: initially provides relief, but dependence can quickly occur. In other circumstances, excessive drinking may produce phobic anxiety. Correct diagnosis again necessary - only possible by withdrawing alcohol, probably in hospital. Avoid temptation to prescribe minor tranquillizers when patient still drinking.

Schizophrenia - not often associated with alcohol abuse; differential diagnosis between schizophrenia and alcohol hallucinosis important. When a schizophrenic patient is abusing alcohol, diagnosis and treatment are necessary in hospital.

Brain damage - brain damage following head injury, cerebrovascular accident or tumour may often lead to alcohol abuse, and these possibilities should always be borne in mind in differential diagnosis.

21

TREATMENT OF ALCOHOL WITHDRAWAL

When a patient is suffering from any mental disorder associated with alcohol, successful management is not possible while the patient is still drinking.

Management of alcohol withdrawal varies with the degree of alcohol dependence and patient's motivation. With only mild symptoms of dependence the patient should be able to abstain without medication but with the support of doctor and family. If medication is required it should never be prescribed while the patient is still drinking.

Either of the following is a suitable treatment regime.

1. Chlormethiazole (capsules 192 mg)

    Day 1   9-12 capsules in 4 divided doses

    Day 2   6-8 capsules

    Day 3   4-6 capsules

    gradually reducing over days 4-6

    Maximum course should last for 9 days. DO NOT PRESCRIBE INDEFINITELY, BECAUSE OF RISK OF ADDICTION
2. Diazepam

    Day 1   10 mg q.d.s.

    Day 2   10 mg t.d.s

    Day 3-4   5 mg q.d.s.

    gradually reducing the dosage over the next 3 days

    Maximum courses should last for 7 days, but smaller doses and shorter courses may be sufficient.

This regime will also be suitable for withdrawal fits.

Parenteral vitamin B supplements (Parentrovite) should be given to prevent the possible development of Wernicke's syndrome and subsequent brain damage.

In treating Delirium tremens, dehydration and electrolyte imbalance must be treated orally. It is difficult to maintain a drip in a delirious patient.

EARLY SIGNS OF ALCOHOL ABUSE

> Excessive spending on alcohol
> Objections from partner
> Neglect of home and family
> Marriage and sexual problems
> Drinking daily, increasing amounts regardless of mood
> Drinking alone
> Poor work record, bad timekeeping, absenteeism
> Frequent surgery attendances for minor illnesses
> Police involvement; Breach of Peace, Drunk Driving
> Frequent excuses for drinking
> Guilt feelings, inability to stop drinking
> Periods of alcoholic amnesia ("blackouts")
> Drinking more and quicker than companions
> Early morning drinking to control withdrawal symptoms

ALCOHOL DEPENDENCE SYNDROME:

"A state, psychic and usually physical, resulting from taking alcohol, characterised by behavioural and other responses that always include a compulsion to take alcohol on a continuous or periodic basis in order to experience its psychic effects and sometimes to avoid the discomfort of its absence: tolerance may or may not be present." (Ninth Revision of the International Classification of Diseases).

Features of the Alcohol Dependence Syndrome:

Narrowing of the drinking repertoire - to relieve or avoid withdrawal symptoms
Priority in maintaining alcohol intake at all costs
Increased tolerance to alcohol
Repeated withdrawal symptoms -
    i.   Tremor - "morning shakes"
    ii.   Nausea and vomiting
    iii. Sweating - early hours of morning
    iv. Mood disturbances
Repeated drinking to avoid withdrawal symptoms
Compulsion to drink associated with loss of control
Return to original drinking pattern after period of abstention

Definitions of "Problem Drinking":

"One who is an excessive drinker, whose drinking causes private or public harm, and who is seen to cause problems for himself or others."
"Intermittent or continuous ingestion of alcohol leading to dependence or harm."
"A person who continues to drink when he has every reason not to do so."
    In practice, few patients present with an "alcohol problem", so that it is very important to be aware of the possibility and look for early signs. As the great mimic in medicine, alcohol is no respecter of persons, and the "Skid Row" pattern is not typical of problem drinkers.

SOCIAL EFFECTS OF ALCOHOL ABUSE

Work - Frequent changes of occupation with reducing responsibility
Increasing periods of unemployment
Occupational hazards; high rate among publicans, actors, seamen, armed forces, journalists, construction workers, medical profession, company directors, sales representatives due to:

23

1. Availability of alcohol
2. Mobility and travel
3. Business entertaining
4. Social pressure to drink
5. Freedom and low supervision

Marriage and family - Increased risk of separation and divorce
        Sexual problems: male impotence and infertility
        Isolation from family: disturbed children

Finances - Increasing proportion of income spent on drinking
        Increased debts and financial difficulties

Housing - Arrears in rent or mortgage repayments
        Standards of housing reduced

Crime - Alcohol-related offences - violent crimes, Breach of Peace
        Drunk driving
        Theft to obtain money

Relationships - Broken friendships
        Narrower social circle, often with other drinkers

Leisure - Few leisure pursuits - "Pool and darts in pub"

PHYSICAL EFFECTS OF ALCOHOL ABUSE

As ethanol circulates freely in the blood stream, no organ is exempt from its effect, although some systems are more obviously affected than others.

Important physical conditions to be borne in mind:

Accidents - Many domestic, industrial and traffic accidents are the result of alcohol excess or abuse, because of impaired coordination and judgment.

Blood disorders - There is a direct toxic effect on the bone marrow. The presence of macrocytosis (MCV>96 fl) is an indication of alcohol abuse. Malnutrition associated with drinking may lead to anaemia.

Chest diseases - Alcoholics have always been prone to chest infections, including pulmonary tuberculosis. Heavy drinking is associated with heavy smoking, hence bronchial carcinoma can be a complication of alcoholism.

Circulatory system disease - Palpitations are a frequent presenting symptom and hypertension is a common sign amongst problem drinkers. Alcoholic cardiomyopathy presents with cardiac enlargement, arrhythmias and heart failure.

Gastrointestinal tract - Symptoms referable to this system are associated with frequent consultations by the drinking patient. Oesophagitis and oesophageal carcinoma are often diagnosed, and gastritis and peptic ulceration are common conditions.

Pancreatitis - An acute abdomen presenting with very severe upper abdominal pain and vomiting; possibly 25% of cases of acute pancreatitis are alcohol-related; the diagnosis can be established by demonstrating a raised serum amylase estimation. Chronic pancreatitis is a complication of alcoholism.

Liver disease - Symptoms of liver disease are vague - general malaise, anorexia, vomiting, upper abdominal pain, with signs of liver enlargement and possibly jaundice. Spider naevi, palmar redness and gynaecomastia may be other signs.

There are three common conditions caused by the toxic effects of alcohol:

a. Alcoholic fatty liver - a reversible condition from which full recovery can take place when the patient abstains from alcohol.
b. Alcoholic hepatitis - evidenced by jaundice, with raised serum bilirubin and transaminases (SGOT and SGTP). Serious complications are hepatic encephalopathy and portal hypertension. Abstension from alcohol can bring full recovery.
c. Alcoholic cirrhosis - Liver tissue becomes necrotic and is replaced with fibrosis, leading to a gradual failure of liver function. Initial enlargement is followed by shrinkage of the organ. This is an insidious, progressive condition later leading to ascites, portal hypertension and oesophageal varices which may bleed profusely. Patients are often impressed by the poor results of liver function tests (raised γ-GTP and bilirubin), and the tangible evidence of liver damage may persuade them to alter their drinking habits. Cirrhosis is an irreversible condition, but abstinence will improve the prognosis.

Peripheral neuropathy - Deficiency of B group vitamins causes degeneration in sensory and motor peripheral nerves. Patients complain of "pins and needles" and "burning feet". Examination reveals absent ankle jerks and diminution in sensation. Adequate treatment with parenteral B vitamins is generally sufficient to produce recovery.

Skeleton - Minor falls may cause fractures; look out for undiagnosed rib fractures. Gout can be a complication of excessive drinking.

An awareness of physical conditions associated with excessive drinking may alert a physician to the possibility of a patient's alcohol problem. It is estimated that as many as 25% of general hospital beds are occupied by patients with alcohol-related illnesses.

MANAGEMENT OF PATIENTS WITH DRINKING PROBLEMS

As patients seldom present with a "drinking problem", the doctor should always be aware of the possibility and should enquire, but not in a censorious manner, about every patient's drinking habits.

To be able to show the patient evidence of the harm his drinking is doing - whether it be physically, mentally or socially - may help to persuade him to alter his ways.

In the first instance, a period of abstinence is always necessary for a full and proper assessment of such physical, mental and social problems that have been caused.

For a patient over 40 years of age, with evidence of physical damage and addiction, and who has failed to control his drinking in the past, future abstinence is essential. The patient should be advised to seek help from Alcoholics Anonymous, local Alcohol Counselling Services and Alcohol Treatment Units if the practitioner feels unable to provide all the support and understanding necessary to help a patient alter his life-style completely.

For younger patients who show no evidence of physical damage, a programme of controlled drinking may be advised, so long as the patient is fully aware of all the risks he runs in abusing alcohol in the future: continuing support will be necessary, for relapses and remissions are unfortunately common.

ALCOHOL

Ethyl alcohol (ethanol) is produced by the fermentation of naturally occurring sugars found in fruit, grain and vegetables, and alcoholic beverages have been in use by mankind from time immemorial. Worldwide, ethanol is regarded as a socially acceptable addictive substance, and alcoholic drinks are used as a condiment with food, as a thirst-quenching beverage and also for religious, ceremonial and social purposes.

Percentage volume of ethyl alcohol in different beverages:

Beers, ciders	4-9%
Wines	9-12%
Fortified wines	17-20%
Spirits	40%

Metabolism of ethanol

Ethanol is readily absorbed from the stomach and small intestine. The most rapid absorption occurs when the volume is 20-30%, and there is also rapid absorption when the drink is effervescent, e.g. sparkling wines or whisky and soda, and when the stomach is empty. The rate of absorption is slowed by the ingestion of food. As ethanol is soluble in water, it circulates freely in the blood stream and reaches all parts of the body, in particular the brain and liver because of their rich blood supply. From 2 to 5% is eliminated unchanged, exhaled by the lungs, excreted by the kidneys and through the skin by sweating. The remainder is broken down in the liver. A healthy liver can only metabolize ethanol at an

26

average rate of 15 mg/100 ml of blood per hour, and this blood level is produced by 8 g(1 cl) of absolute alcohol. This quantity is regarded as a unit of alcohol and is the amount of ethanol contained in:

> 1/2 pint of beer or cider
> 1 glass of wine
> 1 glass of sherry or port
> 1 single measure of spirits

Effects of alcohol on the body

> Small transient increase in heart rate
> Dilatation of skin capillaries producing characteristic flush
> Increased sweating leading to fall in body temperature
> Gastric juices stimulated
> Mild diuretic effect
> Central nervous system depressant, producing disinhibition

Effect of increasing levels of blood alcohol on CNS activity

30 mg/100 ml	Mild feeling of well-being
50 mg/100 ml	Slight unsteadiness
(80 mg/100 ml	Legal limit for driving)
100 mg/100 ml	Obvious ataxia, nystagmus
300 mg/100 ml	Stuporose
500 mg/100 ml	Coma and death

As a guide to "normal drinking", the latest recommendations of the Royal College of Psychiatrists are a total of 28 units of alcohol per week, and a common adage is "2 or 3 pints 2 or 3 times a week".

In view of the rapid increase in alcohol consumption in this country over the past 20 years, and the subsequent increase in all alcohol-related problems, everybody should be advised to halve their present alcohol intake; this would help to minimize the number of patients who will present with alcohol problems in the future.

4

Hallucinated patients

Eric D West

QUICK REFERENCE GUIDE

A. THE DESCRIPTIONS USED

It is unlikely that hallucinations will often be referred to as such. Frequently, in mentally ill patients, hallucinatory experiences are inferred from their behaviour. In alcoholics with delirium tremens the fear reaction may be more apparent than the visual hallucinations. In young children, screaming attacks in the night or nightmares may be described which have a basis in hallucinatory experiences, possibly as a drug reaction or on the basis of a febrile illness.

B. HALLUCINATORY EXPERIENCES

True hallucinations may affect one or more of the senses. Auditory and visual hallucinations are commonest but smell, taste, touch and internal body sensations may be involved. Pseudo-hallucinations may arise in the bereaved where the lost partner may be felt to be still present, but the bereaved person can be persuaded and agree that it is not so, and insight is retained. Hypnogogic hallucinations occur just before falling asleep, and hypnopompic at the threshold of sleep and awakening, and are not usually accompanied by any other behavioural changes. Hallucinations can be induced by hypnosis. Religious hallucinations, visions of God or Christ, may occur in the susceptible, after highly emotional religious assemblies, usually where there are large crowds.

True hallucinations appear to be sensory perceptions, subjectively real to the patient, but not arising from the external or internal environment, e.g. hearing voices in the walls of a house which no one else can hear. Illusions are real sensations which are misinterpreted. Imagery involves reviving a real sense experience, e.g. visualizing a rainbow.

True hallucinations are often combined with delusions in the mentally ill, and generally are associated with behavioural disturbance although they may occasionally be an isolated phenomenon.

C. THE LIKELY POSSIBILITIES

1. In children

A febrile illness, or drugs. The drugs may be prescribed or not prescribed, and may be taken in advised dosage or overdosage. Abuse of solvents is a growing problem. Epilepsy is a possible cause.

2. In young adults

Illicit drugs become an increasing possibility, but reactions to prescribed drugs also occur and overdosage must be considered. In a young person returning from abroad, consider diseases such as typhoid. Mental illness and temporal lobe epilepsy as new cases are relatively infrequent in any one G.P. practice. (Schizophrenia: 18 new cases per 100 000 population per annum.) Schizophrenia presents, on average, 10 years earlier in males than females. Nevertheless, schizophrenia should always be considered.

3. In the middle aged

Consider drugs, alcoholism and mental illness. An infrequent cause could be exposure to industrial toxins, including solvents. Epilepsy, particularly of the temporal lobe should be considered and may have an acquired basis at this age.

4. In the elderly

As with children, the elderly are **more likely to show side effects**, including hallucinations, **to prescribed medication and to illness, particularly infections**. After 70 years of age, and particularly after 80, degenerative brain disease should be considered.

D. REMINDERS: BEFORE SEEING THE PATIENT

Always try to establish the whereabouts of reliable informants. It is sometimes surprising, with the mentally ill, that one particular informant will know all about the details of a patient's symptoms whereas others, perhaps in the same household, will not. In case drug overdose is a problem, look at the record cards of the whole family and note recent prescriptions. A child may have gained access to a parent's or sibling's drugs. Set in motion the obtaining of information from hospitals where relevant. Ask if an industrial or university medical service has been involved.

E. ON SEEING THE PATIENT

After obtaining a history, **establish whether there is clouding of consciousness, including disorientation**. Sometimes patients who will not respond to questions such as: what is the date, the day of the week, etc., will do so when a picture is shown to them, say, of members of the Royal Family; or they will perform a simple task such as matching dominoes for colour and number of dots.

1. With clouding of consciousness, organic factors are more likely.
2. Absence of clouding of consciousness may be difficult to detect in the mentally ill who will not answer questions, but information is usually available on recent behaviour from informants.
3. Concealment of information is frequent in illicit drug taking, alcoholism and mental illness.
4. It is occasionally worth checking the "input from the environment" as a contribution to hallucinations. One mentally ill patient was regarded as having tactile hallucinations because of a sensation of insects crawling on the skin. The diagnosis was revised three weeks later when lice were found in the clothing and louse eggs on hairs. Here a 5X lens proved decisive. Remember, lice stay in the clothing. Scabies still occurs in closed and semi-closed communities.
5. If mental illness, particularly schizophrenia, is suspected, ask to see drawings or writing done by the patient. The existence of bizarre drawings or incoherence or private symbolism in writing may be discovered.
6. In established mental illness check for non-compliance in drug taking - missing depot injections, not taking oral medication.

7. In suspected alcoholic delirium tremens there may be some reason why the patient has not been able to maintain habitual drinking habits, an injury, running out of money or an infection.

F. NON-PRESCRIBED DRUGS AND SUBSTANCES ASSOCIATED WITH HALLUCINATIONS

1. Drugs taken as hallucinogens e.g. LSD (lysergic acid diethylamide) and psylocibin (from mushrooms containing it)

Medical referral is unlikely, but some LSD takers have injured themselves during drug episodes and such conditions as sub-dural haematoma resulting from head injury have occurred and are a possibility to be considered if there is subsequent mental impairment or confusion. "Flashbacks" can occur as psychotic episodes several months after taking LSD. Insight is usually preserved in LSD experiences and it might be more accurate to call the visual experiences pseudohallucinations. LSD cannot be detected biochemically within NHS laboratory services, but as mixtures of drugs are often taken, a general drug profile may be within the scope of the nearest Laboratory Service.

Cannabis in its various preparations can cause perceptual distortions, but again, medical referral is unlikely, although there is sometimes a history of persistent heavy cannabis use before a patient is referred with suspected schizophrenia. It is sometimes difficult to distinguish between schizophrenia which would have occurred in any case and a syndrome with social withdrawal, self-neglect, perceptual distortions which may be a consequence of cannabis use, and at present the relationship is uncertain.

2. Solvent abuse ("glue sniffing") and accidental exposure to industrial solvents

Solvent abuse is maximal in the school age years i.e. the 8-17-year age group, with males outnumbering females by 10 to 1, and may be a group activity and associated with truancy. It is not a criminal offence. Many different substances are involved, petrol, aerosols, dry cleaning fluids, plastic (styrene) cements, model cements, nail polish remover and lighter fluid.

The main toxic constituents inhaled are toluene, acetone, benzene, naphtha, alcohol, trichlorethane and perchlorethylene.

Visual and auditory hallucinations may occur in the induction phase accompanied by euphoria and excitation. Solvent abuse is dangerous. Asphyxiation can occur directly or from inhaled vomit.

(see also p.193).

3. Amphetamines

In prolonged high dosage these can cause a paranoid psychosis with auditory hallucinations which resemble schizophrenia. There may be violent or suicidal behaviour with stereotyped movements. Insight may be gained after withdrawal of the drug.

4. Cocaine

Sometimes used as an adjuvant to heroin taking, also on its own. Tactile hallucinations ("formication") may occur. Recovery with insight on cessation of the drug may distinguish the syndrome from mental illness (see also p.197).

5. Phencyclidine ("Angel dust")

May lead to excitement with dissociation that may be mistaken for true hallucinations.

G. PRESCRIBED DRUGS ASSOCIATED WITH HALLUCINATIONS

Children and the elderly may develop an **acute toxic confusional state** from drugs acting on the central nervous system, from anticholinergic drugs and beta blockers. Cimetidine and digoxin can also be implicated. Digoxin can cause distortion of colour vision, usually yellow vision, which may be mistaken for a visual hallucinatory experience.

In the early stages of toxicity, the level of consciousness fluctuates, with fear and perplexity. In some patients hallucinations may occur, usually visual.

In children recovering from an overdose of tricyclic antidepressants there may be visual hallucinations of red geometrical figures resembling spiders.

In effect, almost any drug can have a "mind-altering-effect" in a susceptible person, but the following could be used as a preliminary check list:

1. sedative drugs used in the daytime or as hypnotics
2. tricyclic antidepressants
3. antihistamines
4. atropine
5. benztropine
6. benzhexol
7. oxprenolol
8. pindolol
9. propranolol

In adults, consider the effects of alcohol, of mixtures of drugs, of the effects of renal or hepatic disease affecting the rate of clearance of metabolites.

Psychotic reactions without clouding of consciousness, sometimes with hallucinations, may occur with:

1. corticosteroids
2. anti-inflammatory drugs such as indomethacin
3. appetite suppressants e.g. diethylpropion and phenmetrazine
4. drugs used in cough mixtures or as antispasmodics such as ephedrine, pseudophedrine, phenylephedrine and salbutamol
5. bromocriptine and levodopa
6. narcotic analgesics e.g. dihydrocodeine and petazocine

In the management of hallucinatory phenomena from drugs, first try to identify the likely offending drug, often difficult with mixed prescriptions and with different doctors involved, including sometimes, on-call agencies where the existing practice records have not been used. Referral to hospital will be the usual course once a preliminary assessment has been made. It is important to try to remain in touch with the patient during the assessment and referral phases, even though rapport may be obtained only in brief interludes.

H. ALCOHOLISM

Two alcoholic states are associated with hallucinations, delirium tremens and alcoholic hallucinosis. In delirium tremens there is clouded consciousness, disorientation, fear, restlessness, tremor, sometimes a raised temperature. Hallucinations may affect any sense but are usually visual and tactile and can be associated with illusions and delusions. Delirium tremens is a medical emergency needing urgent referral to hospital.

Alcoholic hallucinosis involves slight or no clouding of consciousness with restlessness. Persecutory voices are prominent. Psychiatric referral is indicated. Apart from the psychiatric state there may be physical complications of alcoholism (see also Chapter 3).

I. DRUG WITHDRAWAL

Drug withdrawal may lead to confusional states. Barbiturates are now less commonly prescribed. Sudden barbiturate withdrawal can produce a state resembling delirium tremens with delirium, fear and hallucinations. The hallucinatory state following trycyclic antidepressant withdrawal has been already referred to.

J. EPILEPSY

Hallucinations occur, in particular in temporal lobe epilepsy. These
may be visual or auditory or epigastric or olfactory sensations.
Visual hallucinations may be recollected vaguely as unformed, but in
other patients recollection may extend to details e.g. a flock of
seagulls with markings on the birds. Auditory hallucinations may
differ from those in schizophrenia in that instead of voices discussing the patient, they can be primitive sounds such as buzzing, bell-
like sounds, sequences of music or song can occur. Voices can be
heard. Auditory experiences are often associated with vertigo. A
few patients with temporal lobe epilepsy can develop a
schizophrenia-like psychosis thought to be arising from the epileptic
process and not due to the two diseases co-existing. Usually there
is more personality preservation in epilepsy than schizophrenia with
less social withdrawal. The patient to look out for, however, is the
one who develops epilepsy of temporal lobe type later in life, as the
basis might be a space-occupying lesion (see also p.81).

K. HYSTERIA

Hysteria may affect an individual, or be epidemic, usually as short-
lived episodes in girls' schools. In the rare Ganser's syndrome, an
individual may show pseudodementia accompanied by visual and
auditory hallucinations. Religious trance states with hallucinatory
experiences probably involve hysterical mechanisms, but the hallucinations can be coherent with the experience.
  Group hallucinatory experiences have been described in
shipwrecked sailors, which apart from physical deprivations, probably involve hysterical mechanisms (see also Chapter 0).

L. MANIC-DEPRESSION

Hallucinations are not prominent, but if they occur as part of the
illness, they should correspond with the mood state. Remember that
in the elderly depressive, hallucinations may be associated with
drugs used in treatment taken in prescribed dosages or in either
excessive doses or frank overdosage.

M. ORGANIC STATES

Confusional states with or without hallucinations may **present with
"silent" presentations of illness** e.g. apyrexial bronchopneumonia,
infection in collapsed areas of lung secondary to bronchial carcinoma, diabetes, prostatic obstruction with uraemia, myxoedema,
myocardial infarction and pernicious anaemia.
  Patients with Parkinsonism can develop hallucinatory confusional
or psychotic episodes as a **reaction to both dopaminergic drugs**

(e.g. Levodopa) **and anticholinergic drugs** (e.g. benzhexol, benztropine, orphenadrine and procyclidine), and particularly where levodopa is combined with bromocriptine. Parkinsonian symptoms may result from antipsychotic medication, such as the phenothiazines, in addition to the idiopathic and postencephalitic illnesses.

Huntington's chorea may present with schizophrenia-like hallucinations but the other features of the disease distinguish it.

In **early recovery phases from concussion or brain contusion** there may be an episode of confusion with misinterpretation of what is going on around the patient with illusions and hallucinations.

In **vitamin B$_{12}$ deficiency**, in pernicious anaemia, there may be parasthesiae which present as cutaneous hallucinations. Vegans used to suffer from vitamin B$_{12}$ deficiency, but most vegans nowadays are aware of the dangers and use vitamin B$_{12}$ supplements.

In **endocrine and metabolic disorders and in electrolyte disturbances** hallucinations can be part of the picture, e.g. in Cushing's disease and in the several varieties of porphyria.

In **dehydration** due to refusal of food and drink in depression there is usually associated mutism and profound retardation with florid symptoms, such as hallucinations, not evident, but in dehydration with associated mineral salt depletions in general, for example, in post-operative patients, florid hallucinations can develop and increase the difficulty in management.

N. PARANOID STATES INCLUDING PARAPHRENIA

Persecutory states are somewhat ill-defined but as in other conditions in psychiatry, check for clouding of consciousness. Where consciousness is not clouded, or only slightly, check for deafness and reduced visual acuity. In the elderly, hearing aids or glasses may be in the house but are not being used. Paraphrenia is clearly defined in the ninth revision of the International Classification of Diseases as a paranoid psychosis in which there are conspicuous hallucinations, often in several modalities. The personality is well preserved. Mood and thinking disturbances are not the main features (see also p.16).

O. PUERPERAL PSYCHOSIS

This is one of the conditions in psychiatry where there is a danger to the patient and the child and where prompt recognition and action is needed. A number of cases occur within hours or days of discharge from hospital which implies that recognition can be difficult. There is often restlessness and insomnia preceding the florid psychotic episode and the latter can be concealed from hospital staff, although visiting relatives sometimes become aware that all is not well. A patient may become visually hallucinated, seeing an ambulance with flashing lights in the room at the end of the bed and believing it is transmitting messages about the patient or child, perhaps a message that the child is not the patient's or is deformed (see also Chapter 17).

P. SCHIZOPHRENIA

Whereas auditory and visual hallucinations are commonest in schizophrenia, tactile or olfactory hallucinations and disturbed internal bodily sensations also occur. At times, it is difficult to elicit hallucinations in a formal interview, but evidence often accumulates from prolonged observation.

Hallucinations are regarded as part of positive symptoms in schizophrenia, with poverty of ideas, of interests and social withdrawal as part of the negative symptom complex. Hallucinations, therefore, are prominent in initial presentations of the disorder and in relapses.

Hearing voices is the commonest feature. The voices may hold a running commentary on the patient, often critical and defamatory, or they may tell the patient what to do. Patients are often not very explicit about their voices.

At the practical level, active hallucinations are an indication that the schizophrenia may need better control. They may be an indication of non-compliance with treatment, with the need to change the dose or the type of drug used.

Relapse in schizophrenia can follow quite small changes in the patient's circumstances, or some alteration which involves excessive social stimulation or sudden energetic attempts at rehabilitation.

An additional cause of increased hallucinations is excessive use of antiparkinsonian drugs given to offset side effects of antipsychotic medication. Some patients take anticholinergic drugs in quantities above the prescribed dose, perhaps by obtaining prescriptions from both the hospital and their general practitioner, by trading such drugs with other patients, or by appearing for a repeat prescription before the existing one has expired (see also p.18).

Q. SENILE AND PRESENILE DEMENTIA

These patients may be hallucinated as part of their illness, and can easily become so on drug dosages which would not cause such a reaction in a patient without brain disease. Hallucinatory experiences should alert the doctor to episodes of relatively "silent" physical diseases. They may follow slight disturbances in the patient's routine, e.g. in an old lady living alone and partially coping, perhaps partially deaf, hallucinations may develop following a visit of men who have come to repair the television or gas stove. The patient "sees" the men in the house after they have gone.

Antidepressants given for depression or apathy may also cause hallucinatory episodes (see also Chapter 5).

R. SENSORY DEPRIVATION

In formal experiments in which subjects have been deprived of sensory input hallucinatory states have occurred. Outside the experimental situation sensory deprivation can be a partial cause of psychotic symptoms. The exhausted mountain climber, having to spend a night or nights caught in a blizzard or a fog, may become disorientated and hallucinated. More commonly in practice such situations can occur, for example, after cataract operations, but partial deafness may also be present as a contributory factor.

5

Depressed patients

Robert Romanis

QUICK REFERENCE GUIDE

INTRODUCTION

It would be wrong to think of depression as normally seen in general practice as an illness of which crises are a feature: as is the case, for instance, with diabetes or appendicitis. Nevertheless the general practitioner will see a number of emergencies marked by extreme changes of behaviour in the patient, and these will include among others the delirium of congestive heart failure or pneumonia in the elderly, and the bizarre behaviour of hypoglycaemia.

It should also be remembered that in a sense **any** possible **presentation of depression is a minor emergency,** as it may be **the only attempt the patient makes to get help** from the doctor. As will be seen, loss of confidence and a sense of shame at the illness itself are among the diagnostic features, and these make it difficult for the patient to approach the doctor. If this first attempt fails, apart from prolonging the morbidity, the patient may pass more or less rapidly into one of the states we are discussing here as emergencies.

Some of these emergencies will be found to be depressive in origin, and these are now discussed more fully under the heads below.

THE AGITATED PATIENT

The differential diagnosis is from hypomania, acute anxiety or grief, hysteria, drug intoxication, thyrotoxicosis, cerebrovascular accident or cerebral tumour.

Diagnostic features

The patient is tremulous and restless. He may be wandering or even hurrying about the room or the house, unable to settle, constantly shifting position, sitting down and getting up. He may be talking ceaselessly, about his failings, guilt and fears, often with delusions of ill-health, poverty, failure of his marriage and similar ideas. He is very likely to return obsessionally to a subject which may be as far fetched as the proverbial small earthquake in Chile; his attention span for other matters is very short. He may be weeping at least part of the time.

Sleep is bad, and the patient may be totally sleepless. Appetite is typically poor, with the patient sometimes picking at food and sometimes not eating at all. But depressive features are not infrequently reversed, and the younger patient may be eating for comfort, usually sweet or fatty foods.

In **hypothyroidism** the mood is entirely different. The patient will appear bad tempered or exasperated rather than miserable and obsessed, and the preoccupation with pessimistic ideas is absent. There may be characteristic physical signs, though all doctors know, sometimes to their cost, how often exophthalmos or a thyroid swelling or murmur may be absent; but the pulse in agitated depression is most unlikely to be as high as in thyrotoxicosis, and the tremor of depression tends to be coarser and more obvious than that of thyrotoxicosis.

Paradoxically, hypomania may present the greatest difficulty, and is indeed the counterpart of depression; but the manic patient rushes about in an impulsive and apparently positive fashion, unlike the miserable restless hurry of the depressed patient. The manic patient may weep, but his tears are like those of joy or relief. Again, he will be talking, but his conversation is flitting unlike the obsessional perserveration of the depressive, and the subject matter is cheerful, bombastic, self-glorifying and knowing. The depressed patient's talk is pessimistic and guilt-ridden.

Acute grief and anxiety may show many features of the true physiological depression. In anxiety there will be obsessional rumination and in grief there will be guilt. The patient will be difficult of access, and the doctor may well feel some delicacy questioning, say, the recently bereaved patient too closely about his or her

39

own symptoms. If a full history can be taken, criteria for the diagnosis of depression are unlikely to be found, (see below); but in fact the distinction is less important here as the treatment may well be the same as in depressive agitation.

In **cerebrovascular accident** or the occasional acute presentation of **cerebral tumour**, there are likely to be confusion and headache. Headache is rare in depression and though the intellectual retardation of depression may be mistaken for disorientation, closer questioning will show that the patient is apathetic rather than genuinely confused, whereas the patient with cerebral damage is in a shocked state like the post-concussional, and confusion may be total. Above all, there may be localizing signs of cerebral damage, either crude signs in the sensory or motor systems, or subtler distortions of word recognition or object recognition, for instance, or other failures of specific centres regulating cerebral activity.

It is important, and this applies to all cases discussed in this section, that the diagnosis of depression should be a positive one, made on actual symptoms, and not a negative one made merely by exclusion of other diseases. This is of course true of all psychiatric diagnosis, but is perhaps particularly important in the case of depression which has the unfounded reputation of being a vague and ill-defined condition. The criteria for diagnosis are given on pp.43-46.

Management

Deep sedation is the treatment of choice of the grossly agitated patient. It is a question of degree, and light sedation may serve for the less severely agitated. Deep sedation can very rarely be carried out at home: the sedation requires the closest observation, and full nursing care is necessary. The patient's psychiatric state also requires close monitoring. These patients need admission to hospital, and often accept the suggestion readily.

THE WITHDRAWN PATIENT

The differential diagnosis is from schizophrenia, cerebro-vascular accident or tumour, hysteria, and semi-coma, including drug intoxication.

Diagnostic features

The patient is apathetic and immobile but conscious, with normal, if slow, pain reaction and other neurological responses. There may be a history of increasing inactivity, obsession and hypochondria, and neighbours or family may report that the patient has been more and more restricting his movements and concerns. He remains indoors, in a single room or in bed, making no effort to wash, dress, feed or look after himself. He is difficult of access because of his intense self-preoccupation, and if he talks at all it is of guilt, sin and failure, or of discomfort and illness. In elderly patients the slowness and perseveration of talk suggest senile dementia.

The facial expression is miserable, perplexed or bad tempered. In extreme physical retardation, the patient remains immobile and in a physical attitude of despair and hopelessness.

Although entertaining suicidal thoughts, he is too retarded to put these into effect during the most severe stage. The risk increases as clinical improvement allows him to plan and take action before delusions of hopelessness have lifted. Self-neglect and anorexia in these patients are associated with loss of weight. They may become grossly dehydrated, and can starve to death.

Distinction from CVA or the acute appearance of cerebral tumour is by possible neurological signs and by the content of the patient's thoughts, which is relentlessly guilt-ridden, querulous, self-absorbed and hypochondriacal, but without the genuine confusion seen in such neurological cases. The patient is deluded, but not disorientated, except to the extent that he has withdrawn from his surroundings.

The depressive patient's delusions are of guilt, hypochondriasis, ruin or with a paranoid bent, whereas the schizophrenic's themes are usually politics, sex or religion. The withdrawn schizophrenic is likely to be even more difficult of access than the depressive, and his conversation, if any, may show the knight's move in thought and bizarre ideas, contrasting with the obsessional and logical single-track but negative thought of the depressive. Granting the depressed patient's mistaken view of his own health or blameworthiness, his conversation makes some kind of sense: in talking to a schizophrenic one is aware that one has no common premise at all (see also Chapter 2).

Management

Such a patient **must be admitted to hospital urgently**, where ECT is often required. Much persuasion is usually needed as the patient has poor insight and is indecisive to the last degree. It may be necessary to invoke the Mental Health Act, as the risks are high and the prognosis poor for the untreated.

THE SUICIDAL PATIENT

This presents the most obvious emergency of the three. In the former two cases, it may be a matter of degree whether the patient is **alarmingly** agitated or **alarmingly** withdrawn, whereas with the suicidal patient, if an attempt has been made, a change of management is forced upon the doctor.

In practice, **the primary emergency is medical or surgical rather than psychiatric**; the patient may be unconscious, from drugs or from attempted drowning, or bleeding from more than one wound and in need or stitching and transfusion. In either case, the presenting emergency is obvious and **immediate admission to a casualty department is indicated** (see also Chapter 6).

Where the patient has taken an overdose, but is still conscious, the same is true. **The doctor cannot rely on the patient's account** of the dose taken: the patient may be genuinely confused, may have kept no count or may be deliberately out to mislead the doctor; moreover it invariably happens that when an attempt is made to work out how much has been taken from a given receptacle, there is never any record of what was in the receptacle to start with. Where the drug has not yet taken full effect the risk of sudden coma continues for some hours; and it requires gastric lavage followed by several hours of close observation with resuscitation equipment available, before the patient can be considered safe. Even then there may be doubt about exactly what drug the patient has taken.

Although management of the psychiatric emergency usually starts after the suicide attempt has been treated, it should be remembered that determined patients will make a further violent attempt if they remain conscious or when they regain consciousness. For example, one patient threw himself down a stairwell only 15 minutes after a self-inflicted wrist slash had been stitched.

The expressed intention of suicide needs to be taken almost as seriously as the actual attempt. Depressed patients do not bother to lie about suicidal feelings; indeed they may express a fear of "doing something silly"; and the hysteric may well fulfil his threat better than he intends.

Where the suicide attempt has been only threatened, or is obviously trivial, careful judgement is needed in management. Some of these patients need hospital admission as urgently as those who have made more dangerous attempts.

This group will include schizophrenic, hysterical and senile patients, as well as the truly depressed; and the question of how far the persuasion should go, will depend on the diagnosis. Sometimes the patient will have to be admitted under a section of the Mental Health Act; always a painful procedure in the circumstances.

Of these, the true depressed patient will be distinguished by the criteria suggested in these pages, and is probably the easiest to manage. Depressed patients generally have some insight into their condition and are aware of the dangers of suicide, and are sometimes relieved to find that the failed or intercepted suicide has given them a second chance. Many experienced doctors have taken a chance on the rapport they have established with a depressed suicidal patient, and have kept him at home and not been disappointed. But this assumes a fully conscious patient, good rapport, time spent discussing the illness and reassuring the patient, and a good insight on the patient's part.

The prevention of imminent suicide is only possible with an alert 24-hour watch. Even in a psychiatric ward, it is not always possible to prevent the determined suicide.

42

The prevention of the future suicide depends on careful observation. The risk increases:

a. If the condition is getting worse.
b. When a patient passes from a tearful, anxious state to become sullen and withdrawn.
c. When new stresses arise such as unemployment, an intercurrent illness, bereavement, an unwanted pregnancy, material loss or an accident to the patient's family.

Most difficult of all to spot, and in some ways **the most dangerous, is the ending of a period of intense activity in a patient who is, or has recently been depressed.** Such a patient can respond professionally or socially to demands made upon him or her, and may indeed plunge into a spate of work or pleasure to overcome the illness. This is an attempt to produce excitement or arousal, and its sudden ending may be marked by a profound deterioration in the illness. The period of arousal comes to an end when a particular job finishes, when a problem is solved, when the patient goes on holiday, or when the patient reaches the limit of endurance. In these circumstances, sudden and apparently unexpected suicides occur, often when the patient seems at the height of success, having completed some particularly difficult project.

Unhappily, the doctor is not very often going to be aware of all this; but any appeal from the family, any warning that the patient is driving himself or herself desperately, must be taken very seriously.

Antidepressant drugs

These are of little use in a depressive emergency. Their action is slow and their immediate psychotropic effect is nil, although sedative members will correct the sleep pattern quickly. These emergencies need treatment far removed from that of the ordinary depression, where explanation, support and antidepressives of whichever group usually bring the patient back to normal.

PRESENTING SYMPTOMS

It is very important that the doctor should be clear about the definition of depression, and alert to recognize or suspect it as it may deteriorate suddenly into extreme withdrawal or suicide. Any known symptom or problem can be presented in depressive illness, but common ones include:

> Overt depressive symptoms (see below)
> Tiredness
> Bad sleeping
> Loss of sexual desire

43

> Hypochondria uncharacteristic of the patient
> Inexplicable pain
> Uncharacteristic obsession
> Lack of concentration
> Agoraphobia

Or the patient may come wishing to discuss depression, but is afraid or ashamed to; and therefore produces another complaint in the hope that depression may somehow come into the conversation. If a patient says, "I get depressed or fed up about this," it is always worth asking "How depressed? How fed up?" This, and enquiring how the patient is sleeping will often help the patient to open up.

The patient's appearance may be characteristic; one does not often see, even in quite severe cases, the frequently described neglect of shaving and general turnout. But the dull, rather hopeless voice, the glum expression, the sad smile, even the moist eyes, may give a clue, as will the generally gloomy or excessively diffident way of talking.

Once suspicion has been aroused, it is necessary to pursue the following symptoms by tactful questioning. The order given is suggested as the least likely to alarm or antagonize the patient.

CENTRAL SYMPTOMS CHARACTERISTIC OF DEPRESSION

Disturbed sleep pattern

Typically the patient wakes at 1 or 2 am in the depths; less typically, there may be difficulty in getting to sleep for 2 or 3 hours; least typically, the patient oversleeps heavily. An important symptom - patients suffering from recurrent depression often sleep more heavily.

Diurnal variation of the main symptom

Depressed patients usually feel worse in the morning and improve as the day goes on. Younger patients can experience their worst feelings later in the day. Not a very reliable symptom.

Agitation (as described earlier) or retardation

The patient feels unduly tired and is slowed up, in thought, speech and movement. Everything is an effort and indecisiveness is prominent. Memory and concentration are impaired and intent fades so that many patients feel they are going mad. Most important symptoms.

Depressed mood

This may vary from a vague dolefulness expressed as "oh dear, oh dear", to actively suicidal thoughts or actions. In so-called hysterical personalities no mood change is detectable, and the picture is of a smiling depression. A very deceptive picture.

Change in appetite

Decreased in the older patient and even occasionally increased in younger ones.

Change in weight

Not always following the appetite change.

Guilt or self-blame

One can ask, "at your worst, do you find yourself blaming other people, Life with a capital L, or yourself?". The depressed patient will usually admit, sometimes with a rueful smile, that he blames himself and feels unworthy or worthless.

As a criterion of diagnosis, disturbed sleep pattern is the commonest and most reliable change. As mentioned earlier, exceptionally, and curiously enough, depressed mood may not be very prominent.

PERIPHERAL SYMPTOMS

Common in depression, but also found in other illnesses.

1. **Panic attacks**: sometimes brought on by meeting people or other everyday stresses, but often completely spontaneous.
2. **Obsessional rumination**: either over some fancied slight or deprivation, or over shameful memories of the past, often quite slight: an awful thing the patient said to his aunt when he was four.
3. **Hypochondriasis**: undue and uncharacteristic concern by the patient over either his own health, or that of his family.
4. **Phobic states**: both claustrophobia and agoraphobia are found in depression, and may suggest the diagnosis.
5. **Paranoia**. This is one of the many possible points of confusion with schizophrenia. Patients may become grumpy and bad tempered towards their associates; or they may "go off" one particular person or the whole human race. This is more often a sense of dislike rather than the suspicious ideas of reference characteristic of schizophrenia. Patients sometimes feel that

people are looking at them strangely. They may become un-reasonably self-conscious of a large nose or bat ears (see also pp.14,15,16).

6. **Depersonalization.** This is a very common psychic symptom which patients try to describe as giddiness or light-headedness. Most patients agree with the description of full consciousness and awareness, but as if there were a sheet of plate glass separating them from the world.

7. **Loss of self-confidence and pessimism.** These are related to hypochondria, and to the curious selectivity of memory in depression, where the patient remembers only the bad things he or she has done, their failures and their misdeeds, to the exclusion of anything good in their lives.

8. **Physical symptoms.** These include any known symptoms, but particularly pain, usually in the limbs or abdomen; and these often and quite legitimately lead to considerable investigations before the depression diagnosis crosses a doctor's mind.

THE PERSONALITY

The typical depressive personality is tough-minded, self-reliant, hard working, perfectionist, responsible and obsessional. Such a personality is appalled and ashamed at these changes, and often unwilling to talk about them at all. A full and patient history is therefore essential, so the patient may be reassured that this falls into the well-known pattern of organic disease. Most depressive patients respond very well to the hypothalamic explanation of depression, and are particularly impressed with the fact that there is a blood test, however experimental. This sort of explanation is a most effective preliminary psychotherapy, before organic treatment is started.

Even in the severely agitated or deeply withdrawn patient, care-ful questioning will elicit enough of these features, both of per-sonality and of the illness, to determine the differential diagnosis. The hysterical personality is always a problem: but there is a coherence to the depressed patient and his symptoms, even includ-ing his delusions, which is lacking in the more diffuse behaviour of the hysteric. In the same way delusions of the depressed appear as errors of perception, compared with the total unreality of the schizophrenic.

Faced with emergencies of the sort we have described, the doc-tor may feel that fine distinctions of psychiatric diagnosis are out of place: but it is easy for a depressed patient to be labelled schizophrenic, for a schizophrenic to be thought hysterical, and for an hysteric to commit suicide without really meaning to. Suggested guidance is given here at least to separate out the depressives in this tangle of diagnoses.

SUMMARY

Crises are not a feature of depressive illness; but this illness needs to be considered in the diagnoses of three acute emergencies: **the agitated patient, the withdrawn patient and the suicidal patient.**

A. **The agitated patient.** Restless, anguished, phrenetic and importunate behaviour. Differential diagnoses include hypomania, acute anxiety and grief, hysteria, drug intoxication, thyrotoxicosis, cerebrovascular accident or cerebral tumour. Agitated depression carries a relatively high risk of suicide. Management usually requires admission and use of adequate doses of antidepressant and neuroleptic drugs, and often ECT.

B. **The withdrawn patient** who avoids social contacts and obligations and is often slowed up in mind and body. Differential diagnoses include schizophrenia, CVA or tumour, hysteria and semi-coma including drug intoxication. Withdrawn and retarded patients with depressive illness are at risk of failing to eat or care for themselves.

C. **The suicidal patient.** May present as unexpected, inexplicable coma; a badly cut patient may be confused by the doctor with accident or assault.

The immediate emergency is medical or surgical: treatment is for coma, bleeding or asphyxia, and requires immediate admission to casualty.

The first presentation of depression is always a minor emergency as it may be the only attempt the patient makes to see a doctor.

Diagnosis must be positive, based on the recognition of depressive features, not negative, based on the exclusion of other diseases.

The cardinal symptoms of depressive illness:

1. Disturbed sleep pattern.
2. Change in appetite for food.
3. Change in weight.
4. Alteration in level of sexual desire.
5. Diurnal variation of the main symptom.
6. Mood may be depressed, anxious, apathetic, lachrymose or simple well-concealed sadness.

A threat of suicide can never be disregarded, though imminent suicide can only be prevented by a really alert 24-hour watch. The future suicide can be suspected where (1) a known depression is deteriorating; (2) new stresses arise during an existing illness; (3) a period of arousal in the form of a spate of work or pleasure comes to an end. This last is particularly dangerous.

It is important to suspect and enquire for depression in patients presenting with the following symptoms:

> Unexplained tiredness or lethargy
> Bad sleeping
> Uncharacteristic hypochondria
> Inexplicable pain
> Uncharacteristic obsession
> Lack of concentration
> Agoraphobia or claustrophobia
> Panic attacks
> Obsessional rumination
> Hypochondria
> Phobic states
> Paranoia
> Hallucinations
> Depersonalization.

Any of the symptoms listed below.
Loss of self-confidence, pessimism and an undue effect of gloomy news. Physical symptoms.

In the three emergencies we are considering, tactful and patient questioning will elicit enough information to decide whether a true depressive illness is present or not.

6

Suicide and parasuicide

Alan Poole

QUICK REFERENCE GUIDE

THE SORTING PROCESS

In attending those who present a threat or who have attempted self harm, consider all to be potentially suicidal until proved otherwise. Wherever possible base your diagnosis on fact illicited by careful enquiry of those who know the patient, evaluation of the history he gives and your examination of him.

Is the threat associated with an obvious change of character or general behaviour?

A. Obvious change

1. If it is associated with a change in sleep, appetite, weight, interest and enthusiasm for work, recreational and sexual activity (biological features), consider affective psychosis.
2. If it is associated with recent major social or personal relationship changes, consider adjustment reaction or onset of affective psychosis.

3. If associated with recent or active physical illness, consider symptomatic depressive psychosis or administration of steroid hormones.
4. If associated with confusion, delirium, hallucinosis or distortion of perception, consider illicit drug taking - amphetamine, cocaine and hallucinogens like LSD.
5. If the biological features are absent but delusions, hallucinations, particularly auditory, or incongruity of affect are present, consider schizophrenia.

B. Without obvious change in character or general behaviour but:

1. With a consistently pessimistic outlook and depressed mood, consider depressive personality disorder.
2. With exaggerated, theatrical behaviour, consider histrionic personality disorder.
3. With sentimental emotionality, memory impairment and facies, consider chronic alcoholism.
4. With intimidation, threat or aggressiveness, consider sociopathic personality disorder.

It goes without saying that the doctor called to one who has harmed himself for whatever reason will attend to the physical care of his patient immediately. Here consideration is given to the diseases and processes which lead to deliberate self harm or remain following an unsuccessful attempted suicide. Self destruction is as abnormal as death from physical disease. There is always a motive for it though the motive itself may be morbid as when acting upon a delusion. Altruistic suicide is an exceptionally rare event.

Stengel defined a suicidal act as any deliberate act of self damage which the person committing that act would not be sure to survive. Hence a parasuicidal (para = beside, beyond or irregular) act is any deliberate act of self damage which the person committing that act believes he will survive. It is the antithesis of suicide in the sense that it is motivated by reasons which appear to the perpetrator to improve his state of well being by the use of an ultimate coercive means. By mistake or ignorance a parasuicidal attempt may end in death; by mistake or ignorance a suicidal attempt may end in survival. The threat of either, whether stated openly or considered a likely component of a disease process, must be taken seriously. Diagnosis can rarely be made simply be examination of the patient. A knowledge of premorbid personality is essential; unless the doctor has it, he must question informants.

DISEASE PROCESSES WHICH MAY LEAD TO SELF HARM

1. Affective psychosis

Depressive illness is the commonest cause of suicide. In this context it matters little whether the cause is reactive or endogenous. It may present with suicide or attempted suicide but nearly always there are **indications of pathological changes of behaviour beforehand**. Normal character features colour the presentation of these signs and symptoms; the stoic conceals them and the histrionic exaggerates them but there is always evidence of **pessimism, apathy and disinterest** in duties, hobbies and recreations. The patient may lack enthusiasm for the future or even deny its existence. There is a preoccupation with unhappy past events which are normally forgotten. **Guilt is always present**. A plausible reason or frank delusion may be offered as explanation. In severe cases the patient may claim that his body or mind are decaying or are in some way harmful to others. **Physical symptoms are common** and when reassured that nothing is amiss the patient's gloom deepens, particularly if he is told that his complaints are imaginary. Frequently they are sensations caused by autonomic dysfunction. The patient may develop **derogatory auditory hallucinations**. Anxiety with restlessness of mind and body is common in the elderly. In other cases retardation is prominent. Slowing of mental processes produces **the appearance of dementia** (depressive pseudo-dementia). The patient may become constipated; sexual libido declines. Secondary amenorrhoea occurs and men cease to experience erection on waking. There is a change in the number of hours spent asleep. **Commonly insomnia occurs** but paradoxically in some young persons and adults having personality traits which mimic youthfulness, sleep may be increased. **Appetite and weight changes** accompany sleep disturbance. Most commonly they are diminished and are sometimes profound, arousing the suspicion of chronic physical illness or malignancy. When an individual experiences hypersomnolence, the appetite is increased and body weight gained.

Melancholic mood is erroneously considered central to the diagnosis of depressive illness. It may exist but be extremely well concealed by those who have been nurtured in the tradition of the "stiff upper lip" and who are naturally unemotional. Evaluation has to encompass the concordance (congruity) of the mood with the content of thought as expressed. In suicidal depression the happiest abstract topics, if considered at all, attract a mood of unhappiness. The patient must always be questioned about suicidal ideas and intent. Unfortunately the answers can be misleading. Middle-aged men, those most likely to kill themselves, will conceal their intention and the histrionic will make melodramatic claims which lack seriousness. Far greater **weight should be placed on presuicidal patterns of behaviour such as visits to priest, solicitor and bank manager, evidence of "setting one's house in order"**.

Suicide may occur in the variant of hypomania known as the mixed affective state. In this condition there are rapid fluctuations of mood. A change from elation to depression may take a matter of minutes. The presence of elation prevents suicidal intent being spotted.

2. Schizophrenia

There is a higher incidence of suicide in those diagnosed schizophrenic than in the general population. Those most **vulnerable** are usually young adults **in the early stages of the illness** who are aware that their mental processes are undergoing serious change. Such individuals are usually socially isolated and experiencing strained relations with parents or friends. They show delusions, hallucinations, thought disorder and inappropriate (incongruous) affect. Special mention must be made of the late paraphrenic form of this illness. It afflicts those in late middle age or the senium who throughout their lives have tended to reclusiveness. Bereavement may increase their isolation. Delusions are florid, persecutory and derogatory in nature. Biological features of affective illness are absent and other aspects of character remain relatively intact. Such patients may take their lives either as a consequence of the nature of their delusions or in a depressed mood caused by them.

3. Neurotic and personality disorders

Although parasuicidal behaviour is associated with these conditions it must be remembered that affective illness can occur coincidentally. In some cases, such as the highly conscientious, pedantic anankast, the character state appears to increase vulnerability to depressive illness. **The clue to diagnosis lies in the presence of the biological features of disturbed sleep, appetite and libido.** The conspicuous neurotic or personality trait colours the presentation and may, unfortunately, obscure its severity and cause suicidal deterioration to be overlooked. Considerable caution should be exercised when one of previously balanced character attempts suicide or makes a parasuicidal gesture in response to trivial provocation or the act itself is puerile in manner. This is very frequently a symptomatic character change caused by organic brain disease. Those of true histrionic character present a real challenge in assessment of suicidal intent. They present their emotions in theatrical manner, with emphasis. They tend also to be of irregular habits hence correct evaluation of sleep and appetite patterns may be difficult.

4. Acute reactions to stress

Increasingly one sees patients of balanced character who respond to stress by parasuicide. Most **frequently the stress is jilting, marital breakdown or to avoid criminal proceedings.** There is a clear and

52

obvious motive which the patient makes little real attempt to conceal. **The timing, place and manner of the act gives a clear indication of the intention.** When presented with such a problem the doctor should retain objectivity and it is surprising how frequently after a short lapse of time in secure hands and with simple counselling the patient recovers composure and stability.

Acute bereavement reactions are quite different. **The diagnostic features of depressive illness are present,** feelings of guilt and self recrimination are strong and the patient shows an insatiable desire to recapitulate the events and feelings associated with the death which taxes the most sympathetic relative. Frequently the situation is made worse because the patient has endured prolonged sleep deprivation whilst engaged in terminal nursing care. **Such patients are particularly vulnerable to impulsive suicidal or parasuicidal acts** (see also Chapter 12A).

5. Organic states

Incidence of death by suicide is particularly high in those suffering from Huntington's Chorea and other presenile dementias. The act takes place during the stage of the disease when awareness is retained at least to some degree. Although the features of depressive illness may be present, this is not always the case. Alzheimer's Disease may present as a depressive illness.

Suicidal depression can be precipitated by virus infections, typhoid fever, brucellosis and tuberculosis and by the therapeutic use of **steroid hormones and ACTH.** It may complicate Cushing's syndrome and acromegaly. Histrionic behaviour with episodes of self harm are associated with **parathyroid disease.**

Acute over-indulgence in alcohol and cannabis, which has a similar effect, induces disinhibition and tips the vulnerable into suicide or parasuicide. In the long term depressant drugs like **alcohol and barbiturates,** particularly during withdrawal, **induce states of melancholy and suicidal pessimism.** The established alcoholic becomes maudlin and prone to self destructive impulses in gloom.

Withdrawal of amphetamines and cocaine induces profound depression complicated by persecutory delusions and fluctuating psychomotor agitation. This is a dangerous situation as is intoxication with LSD and other hallucinogens which cause confusion, distortion of perception, hallucinosis and exaggerated emotional states.

Increasingly doctors are exposed to the direct threat that unless they accede, usually the prescription of drugs, the patient will take his life. It is folly to be tempted to act contrary to the best clinical interests of the patient. Courage is required in saying no convincingly. Specialist treatment is preferable to controlled abuse.

Finally, situations which require particular caution because of the risk of suicide

1. The depressed man in his fifth or sixth decade of life, particularly those of social standing and responsibility.
2. The patient who is improving from severe retarded depressive illness and has reached the stage of recovering initiative and drive. This could be during premature trial leave from hospital treatment.
3. The patient who has experienced prolonged sleep disturbance, whether as part of a depressive illness, physical illness, caring for a sick relative or unusually prolonged night shift work.
4. In those with pain syndromes, physical or hypochondriacal complaints or delusions who have failed to be reassured that there is nothing amiss.
5. A previous history of suicide attempt of a nature or in a situation which would leave little or no possibility of intervention.
6. Those who admit suicidal thoughts or intentions only with great reluctance and are known to have made recent provision for dependants (see also pp.18,100,118).

7

Hysterical patients

Joan Gomez

QUICK REFERENCE GUIDE

The diagnosis of hysteria is denigrated by some authorities and as passionately defended by others. The family clinician has no doubt of its existence in practice and the International Classification of Diseases, Ninth Revision recognizes 8 subtypes of hysteria, hysterical personality and the related disorders: Briquet's syndrome and hypochondriasis.

ESSENTIAL CHARACTERISTICS OF HYSTERICAL SYMPTOMS:

- produced - or maintained - by psychogenic mechanisms of which the patient is unaware
- consistent with patient's own concept of physical, sensory and psychological functioning in illness
- likely to attract lay and also medical concern
- related to emotional conflict which may not be obvious

Other likely features:

- cause immediate reduction of anxiety: primary gain for example, losing one's voice before giving an (ill-prepared) lecture
- secondary gain: through indulgence or gratifying interest from others, and facilitation of manipulating the situation
- symbolic choice of symptoms, for instance a middle-aged man was struck blind when he came upon his wife in bed with her lover
- "belle indifference": inappropriate equanimity in the face of apparently ominous symptoms. Some patients show instead extreme anxiety and persistent, often angry demands for relief.

The existence of indubitably hysterical symptoms does not, of course, remove the possibility of concurrent disease: hysterical symptoms are common at the onset of a schizophrenic episode, in epileptics, in the presence of neurogical disorders including organic brain syndromes, and with malignancy anywhere. On the other hand, proven organic disease does not prevent the development of hysterical symptoms: in epilepsy, for example, genuine and psychogenic fits may both occur.

VULNERABILITY FACTORS

- immaturity of personality, especially sexually, at any age, either sex, and whatever intellectual status
- passivity, dependence, suggestibility
- immigrant or other non-dominant status, for instance female members of Asian or Middle Eastern families
- experience of illness, either direct or vicarious, for instance father frequently unable to go to work because of back pain
- illness-rewarding situation, for instance increased attentiveness of bored husband or being excused from heavy work
- organic brain damage in early childhood: birth and later trauma, meningitis etc
- recent minor head injury
- previous hysterical symptoms, or unexplained symptoms, or unexplained symptoms which recovered undiagnosed, for instance 8 months' aphonia following a mugging incident
- genetic factors in Briquet's syndrome only
- communication difficulties: language problems, lack of verbal skill (unrelated to quantitative output), lack of perception and receptiveness by others

TYPES OF PATIENT TO BE CONSIDERED IN DETAIL:

Those with hysterical personality
Hysterical neurotics: with symptoms presenting in the following systems:

- neurological: dissociative and conversion symptoms
- gastrointestinal
- gynaecological/genitourinary
- cardiorespiratory
- musculoskeletal
- dermatological
- psychiatric

Suffers from epidemic or culturally-determined hysterical syndromes
Briquet's syndrome
Hypochondriasis
Patients with persistent pain - at least in part psychogenic
Children with hysterical symptoms
(Munchausen's disorder and other forms of malingering)

HYSTERICAL OR HISTRIONIC PERSONALITY
(also described in Chapter 21, Moodiness, page 222)

Features: it occurs most often in women and some artistic and homosexual men with a streak of submissiveness in their make-up. It can be a normal personality type, frequently found in the acting profession, and comprising extraversion, sociability and helpfulness. Such people are charming and entertaining companions: albeit at a superficial level. They like to be centre-stage, or failing that, in the entourage of some idol, accommodating to his every whim.

Morbid hysterical emotionality, by contrast, causes suffering to others. The patient manipulates them into situations which provide an outlet for dramatic scenes - of self-pity, temper, demands for proof of love, threats of self-injury, panic and also displays of affection and sexuality. The patients' need for constant change and novelty leaves their partners bewildered. Only too easily extravagant devotion is replaced by spite and accusations: the doctor may be on the receiving end.

Management: skill and flexibility are required. These patients combine flattery, seductiveness, both intellectual and sexual, and gifts - in a matrix of dependency and demands for special treatment, often the impossible. Frustration and perceived rejection are likely to result in an angry reaction, for instance overdosage or a complaint about the doctor to the authorities. Medication usually has no - safe - place in the treatment of hysterical personality: what is needed is a reliable, regular, limited investment of time for discussion with the patient. Hysterical dissociation or conversion symptoms are only slightly more prevalent in those of hysterical personality than in others.

Dissociative phenomena: these comprise disorders of memory, consciousness and intellect and represent a splitting off from the field of awareness a part that includes something threatening or distressing to the patient. They appear as neurological or psychiatric symptoms.

Conversion phenomena: these are disturbances of function in any system or part of the body, which are produced by the transformation of emotional states or mental conflicts without the patient's being aware of their origin. Such psychogenic symptoms include pains, paralyses, tremors, spasms, vomiting, blindness or fits - and others.

NEUROLOGICAL PRESENTATIONS

Psychogenic amnesia: typically the patient is found, apparently lost, and brought to a hospital, police station or doctor's surgery by a kind passer-by. Sometimes the patient herself (or himself) presents and asks for help, quite calm but unable to give an account of herself apart from the last half hour or so. Occasionally hysterical amnesia refers only to a circumscribed period and cluster of events, but usually it involves the blotting out of large parts of the patient's life, including her personal identity. Consciousness is unclouded and there is a general preservation of mundane information and intellectual abilities. The patient can read, write, operate the telephone or interpret a proverb: unless the questions are perceived as a test.

Hysterical fugue: some patients who develop amnesia come to notice within a few hours but others wander to some distance from where they are known or from an unpleasant situation. This type of fugue may last for days or weeks (see Table 1).
  A typical stressful backdrop to the development of hysterical amnesia is a sexual adventure in a schoolgirl or young wife, who dare not go home. In men it is more often a broken bail or probation order in another area.

Multiple personality: this is a rare variant of the fugue state - when it is genuine - in which the patient, through suggestion, intentional or otherwise, takes on a different personality from his own for all or part of the time. More often it is a matter of deliberate pretence for gain, as in the case of Bianchi, the American multiple murderer who assumed 3 different personalities while he was in custody.

Management of psychogenic amnesia: in most cases memory returns spontaneously within hours or a few days in a supportive environment, and once started recovery is rapid. Meanwhile enquiries about missing persons may be made from the police and psychiatric hospitals: in hysterical cases the patient carries no cards, letters or

Table 1 DIAGNOSTIC FEATURES IN FUGUE STATES

	PSYCHOGENIC Hysterical fugue	ORGANIC Transient global amnesia	Post-ictal automatism
Sex	F more than M	M more than F	Either
Age	Commonly 15-40	50+	Any
Duration	Hours, days occasionally weeks	4-8 hours	Minutes - hours
Precipitants - physical	Head injury or alcohol sometimes precede	Usual, e.g. vascular	Not usually
- emotional	Usually	Occasionally	Not relevant
Behaviour	Co-ordinated, despite seemingly aimless wandering	Normal	May be stereotyped or purposeless
Appearance	Adequately cared-for	As usual	Dishevelled
Personal identity	Cannot recall	Preserved	Preserved
Conscious level	Normal	Normal	Impaired
Affect	Bland or depressed	Perplexed	Fearful
Electro-encephalogram (EEG)	Normal	Abnormal	Abnormal/epileptic

Note: "delayed concussion" is a favourite lay explanation for hysterical fugue, but this is not borne out by medical experience. However it is not uncommon for a minor head injury to precede a hysterical fugue for which there are emotional reasons.

other easy means of identification. Immediate restoration of memory may be induced by a slow intravenous injection of amylobarbitone sodium to induce relaxation, not sleep, usually requiring less than 250 mg. The sudden flooding-back of anxiety-laden memories may be intensely distressing and even lead to a suicidal attempt. It is kinder and safer to arrange for the patient to remain in a psychiatric facility for a few days while her memory returns as she feels more secure. Small daily doses of diazepam - 2 mg t.d.s. - ease the process. If memory does not recover within about 4 days it is likely that hysterical amnesia has merged into malingering.

After return of memory neurotic depression may remain. It is best treated by supportive discussion. A full explanation of how the time of the fugue was spent is not usually forthcoming, nor should the details be sought.

Stupor: this condition is characterized by complete or almost complete absence of spontaneous movement and speech, although twitching and muttering may occur. The patient is unresponsive to most

Table 2 DIAGNOSTIC FEATURES IN STUPOR

	Hysterical stupor	Catatonic state	Organic stupor

Past history:
  Neurological
  Psychiatric
	
	-
	+
		
		-
		+
			
			+
			-

Response to dropping patient's arm above his face	Avoids nose	Waxy flexibility: arm stays up	No attempt to protect face
Resistance to passive movement	May be ++	Waxy flexibility or resistance +	None
Personally stressful situation	+	-	-
Waxing/waning of stupor	+	-	-
Autonomic arousal, e.g. rapid pulse	++	+	-
Mention of emotive subjects leads to increased pulse rate	+	-	-

Eye signs:
  Blepharospasm
  Rapid closure after forcible opening
  Doll's eye reflex
	
	+
	+
	
	-
		
		-
		-
		
		-
			
			-
			-
			
			+ (if the head is moved, both eyes turn to other side)

Eyes deviate towards ground with pt lying on either side	+	+	-
Gaze wanders	-	-	+
Equal, dilated, responsive pupils	+	+	Maybe
Co-ordinated response to painful stimuli	+	±	-

stimuli, implying impairment of consciousness, but there may be indications that the patient is after all aware of what is going on. His
eyes may be open, and appear watchful, but are more often closed
in hysterical types of stupor (see Table 2).

Depressive stupor, which usually develops through increasing retardation in a depressive illness, resembles catatonic (schizophrenic)
stupor apart from the absence of waxy flexibility. Possible organic
causes include uraemia, myxoedema, hypoglycaemia, hepatic disorders, alcohol and other intoxications, as well as more serious
cerebral disorders: most important is raised intracranial pressure.
Neurological signs will be evident.

Management of hysterical stupor: reassuring talking to the patient, despite apparent lack of response for some time; physical support; wait and observe. Small doses of diazepam by any route may help. Obviously admission must be arranged if recovery is delayed more than an hour or two.

Hysterical seizures: pseudo-epileptic fits are the second commonest manifestation of hysterical disorder: the situation is compounded by the occurrence of hysterical fits in patients who also suffer genuine grand mal attacks (see Table 3).

Table 3 DIAGNOSTIC FEATURES IN SEIZURES

HYSTERICAL	EPILEPTIC (see also p.34)
Colour normal, flushed or pale	Cyanosis or pallor
May moan or scream	One initial cry or nothing
Never in sleep or alone	May be when asleep or alone
Thrashing movements, trunk involvement	Tonic-clonic pattern
Variable awareness	Unconscious
Injury and tongue-biting rare	May occur, signs of old injuries common
Incontinence rare	Urinary incontinence common
Corneal reflex retained	Absent during seizure
After fit	
Normal plantar response	Extensor plantar response
Normally reactive pupils	Dilated unresponsive pupils
May complain of confusion	Confusion and sleep follow fit
Tests: EEG always abnormal in grand mal	
Serum prolactin usually raised after grand mal fit	

One-third of patients who have hysterical fits also have epilepsy; the others have nearly always had vicarious experience - in their families or at work.

Management of hysterical fits: check that patient cannot inadvertently hurt herself but **do not restrain** movements - this enhances them. After fit develop rapport with patient and help her and her (or his) relatives to gain insight. Discuss emotional difficulties with interviews at increasing intervals over about 18 months. If the patient is clinically depressed treat by psychotherapy if possible: avoid maprotiline. Paradoxical treatment may be undertaken with relatives' consent and cooperation: the patient rests in a darkened room with minimal stimuli. Restrictions are gradually lifted as fit-free intervals lengthen, and psychotherapeutic discussions then proceed.

Pseudo-status epilepticus: although hysterical fits often have a greater frequency than true grand mal, pseudo-status is rare. In genuine status the seizures are separated by intervals of not more than 15-30 minutes, becoming progressively shorter and less vigorous. Thrashing about does not occur. Consciousness is not restored between fits.

Pseudoepilepsy resembling simple partial seizures of the motor type: the hysterical patient may show twitching on one side of the face, or jerking of the limbs on one side. There may be trembling and irregular shaking. In an organic focal fit the movements are either clonic or tonic and seldom affect the shoulder or elbow without involvement also of the face and hand. In a right-sided motor seizure speech is arrested in genuine epilepsy. Treatment of hysterical cases is as for other hysterical fits (see above).

Hysterical faints, falls and dizziness:

Hysterical faints: differ from syncope in that the typical onset is lacking: nausea, weakness, yawning, sweating, epigastric discomfort. There may be pallor, but there is no bradycardia, no hypotension, and the patient is likely to remain unresponsive for more than a few seconds. No reflex flushing occurs. The patient is always in the erect posture at the onset of syncope except in the unusual "supine hypotensive" syndrome in pregnancy.
Management: the hysterical faint expresses upset or insecurity and needs reassurance.

Falls without loss of consciousness: in the young especially, transient "giving way" of the legs is likely to be hysterical, but in the elderly may be due to transient ischaemia in the distribution of the vertebrobasilar artery. Cataplexy - sudden loss of muscle tone - may be associated with narcolepsy. However "narcolepsy" itself may often be a hysterical manifestation: a child may be unrousably asleep when it is time to go to school unlike true narcolepsy in which the patient may fall asleep at a banquet - with his face in his plate of food.

Dizziness: psychogenic dizziness is difficult to describe and is usually part of a mix of symptoms. It lacks the sensation of rotation of vertigo, and is not usually experienced as like flying or falling, as in delirium and other organic disorders. Dizziness, possibly hysterical in some cases, is part of the post-traumatic syndrome, accompanied by headache. Orthostatic hypotension and the effects of hyperventilation may also induce organically a feeling of dizziness, as may cardiac disorders, and certain drugs: tricyclic antidepressants, MAOIs, phenothiazines particularly.

Neurological disorder presenting as hysterical conversion symptoms

Certain organic neurological disorders predispose to hysterical conversion, for instance:

> multiple sclerosis
> epilepsy (vs)
> focal abnormality in the temporal lobes
> mental retardation
> toxic/metabolic encephalopathies
> encephalitis
> brain tumour

These should be remembered as a possible backdrop to hysterical symptoms.

MOTOR DYSFUNCTION

Weakness and paralysis: paralysis of the tongue, extraocular muscles and face does not occur through hysterical mechanisms, and it is rare for there to be hysterical paresis of the cervical muscles. The trunk musculature is seldom involved - so it is the limbs which are most often affected. Hysterical disorder impairs movements rather than individual muscles or muscle groups. Typically, on passive movement the limb gives way discontinuously and the antagonist muscles may contract, exaggerating apparent weakness. If a "paralysed" limb is held up and released, in hysterical cases it will hover a second or two before falling, indicating some muscle tension. A great show of effort may be made if, for instance, the patient is asked to squeeze two fingers.

Hemiplegia: hysterical mechanisms may be demonstrated by asking the patient to raise his "good" leg, while holding one's hand under the heel of the affected side: pressure downwards occurs if the paralysis is psychogenic. Neurological signs will be absent.

Astasia-abasia: - hysterical gait - leads to falls when the patient may be observed, but injury is trivial. The affected leg is dragged rather than swung round as in organic hemiplegia. Clutching, staggering and even crawling are displayed without embarrassment. However, the frontal lobe (organic) syndrome should be considered: in this both gait and affect are odd, and urinary incontinence is common.

Muscular rigidity: if this is hysterical it increases in proportion to the effort made by the examiner to move the part. Warning - this also occurs in dystonia: involuntary, slow, sustained, contorting movements of organic origin, and also in the frontal lobe syndrome.

Tremor: the hysterical type is coarse and irregular, lacking the rhythmicity of Parkinsonism. Diagnostic doubts are likeliest with tremor due to lithium toxicity. Unfortunately organic tremor worsens with stress as does the hysterical, and on intention if it is cerebellar.

Aphonia and dysphonia in which the voice is too soft or hoarse for effective communication is likely to be hysterical if it comes on suddenly in a young, fit person, especially female, following an emotive event. A girl who was attacked in the street found she could not scream at the time - nor speak for 6 months afterwards. She had been terrified of being knifed if she made a noise. Sometimes aphonia protects the patient from letting out some indiscretion or legal peccadillo.

Ocular symptoms: blepharospasm in the middle-aged may be due to rare, progressive neurological disease, but is commonly hysterical in the absence of obvious local trouble. A woman patient, bored by her mundane marriage, developed blepharospasm in the evenings, preventing her from cooking her husband's supper, or indeed from seeing him.

Diplopia if monocular, and **tunnel vision** that does not widen out with increasing distance are likely to be hysterical. Post-traumatic issues sometimes operate in these cases. Muscle spasms and stiffness are considered under musculo-skeletal symptoms (see below).

SENSORY DYSFUNCTION

Anaesthesia or paraesthesiae of hysterical origin are usually clear-cut in distribution conforming to the precise midline or for instance, glove or stocking area. The patient may do up a button or tie a lace without clumsiness if his loss of sensation is hysterically determined.

Hysterical blindness is likely to arise suddenly in the context of injury or emotional shock: pupillary reactions are unaffected, unlike the situation in organic cases apart from occipital lesions.

Hysterical deafness, partial or complete, does not prevent the patient being woken by a noise nor reacting to an unusual or emotive sound behind him.

Management of conversion symptoms in general is dealt with later but it is of particular relevance in neurological presentations to identify the primary benefit or relief afforded by the particular dysfunction. **WHAT CAN THE PATIENT NOT NOW DO - OR SAY, HEAR, FEEL OR SEE - THAT WOULD OTHERWISE HAVE BEEN EXPECTED?** Secondly, however clear it is that the symptom is not, after all, organically based, the patient's dignity must be preserved. **HE MUST BE ALLOWED TIME IN WHICH TO ADJUST AND RECOVER AND AN EXPLANATION THAT IS NOT HUMILIATING.**

GASTROINTESTINAL PRESENTATIONS

-   dysphagia, including "globus hystericus": MAY have an organic cause in the neurological system, apart from obvious local pathology. Many cases reflect emotional, often sexual conflict.
-   vomiting - without organic basis - is common in young women: expressing ambivalent feelings towards parents, husband or sexual activity. It may be part of anorexia nervosa.
-   abdominal pain, heartburn: may be a symptom of depression or of mental conflict.
-   anorexia, with or without weight loss.
-   nausea: hysterical causes are usually easily discovered - what repulses the patient?
-   fulness, bloating: often associated with aerophagy.
-   anorectal burning, irritation: may reflect sexual guilt or a desire to be rid of someone.
-   bulimia, constant thirst: if functional, likely to represent lack of emotional fulfilment.
-   diarrhoea, constipation: if psychogenic more commonly associated with chronic tension than hysteria.

GYNAECOLOGICAL/GENITOURINARY PRESENTATIONS

These are particularly common as part of Briquet's syndrome (see below).

-   pelvic pain: often following pelvic inflammatory disease.
-   dyspareunia, vaginismus: often based on doubts about the integrity of the partner, or fear of pregnancy.
-   penile pain, erectile failure: guilt or ambivalent feelings about the partner; fear of responsibility.
-   anaesthesia of genital area: usually in women who, after childbirth or hysterectomy, dislike the thought of intercourse, and are anyway irritated by their partner.
-   pseudocyesis: manifest in amenorrhoea, abdominal distension, nausea and breast sensations: usually in older, childless women, but sometimes a reflection of guilt in a younger one. The umbilicus remains dimpled.
-   urinary retention: usually in a young woman, who is unconcerned and shows no signs of acute discomfort.
-   burning or itching in the genital area: often associated with unacknowledged anger towards the partner, less often guilt over an indiscretion.
-   amenorrhoea, menstrual irregularities: these may occur with any neurosis or psychosis, or through hysterical mechanisms in emotional conflict.

CARDIORESPIRATORY PRESENTATIONS

- chest pain: most often in men, sometimes but not necessarily after myocardial infarction: to escape unwanted activity, either work, sexual or menial.
- palpitations: often part of Briquet's syndrome, and arouses concern in others.
- cough, throat-clearing: indication of complaints the patient dare not air - against employer, nearest and dearest.
- dyspnoea: expressing fear and an inability to cope.
- breath-holding: common in young children in a rage with an important other person, which they cannot or dare not express.

MUSCULOSKELETAL PRESENTATIONS

- torticollis, hemifacial spasm, writer's cramp - may all appear to be hysterical yet can prove to have a neurological basis. However, spasm of the adductor muscles of the thighs in a young girl is likely to be hysterical, as is the painful spasm of the fingers in an instrumentalist who is over-anxious about his performance.
- stiff, painful joints: in someone with vicarious experience of arthritis and a longing to be looked after rather than do unwanted chores, commonly. Back pain may have a hysterical aetiology, or reflect depression or tension.
- tics and twitches may be hysterical or symptomatic of high tension rather than conflict and the hope of relief.

DERMATOLOGICAL PRESENTATIONS

- blushing, itching and burning: depending on the area affected may have a different symbolic meaning - but basically express a sense of danger and insecurity in relationships.
- dermatitis artefacta: the patient denies and is probably unaware of the damage he or she inflicts on his skin. Most such patients have disturbed social backgrounds and personality problems of some standing.

PSYCHIATRIC PRESENTATIONS

Psychogenic production of psychiatric symptoms seems almost a contradiction in terms, but the same underlying mechanisms apply. The apparent illness is the best answer the patient can come up with in an intolerable situation. Among such situations may be an incipient functional psychiatric illness such as depression or schizophrenia, or an organic brain syndrome, acute or chronic.

Hysterical pseudodementia: this needs differentiating not only from organic dementia but the depressive variety (see also Chapter 15). Features:

-   common antecedents are rows at home, money troubles, legal or disciplinary problems, sexual complications.
-   the patient may have wandered off and can give no explanation.
-   previous head-injury with unsettled compensation issues may be a factor.
-   mute, monosyllabic or grossly incoherent.
-   self-care and eating habits unimpaired.
-   inconsistent performance, influenced by suggestion.
-   apparently disorientated but does not perseverate, and does not give concrete interpretations of proverbs.

Unlike depressive states, appetite is normal, mood not markedly miserable, nor is retardation a feature.

Ganser's syndrome: this was considered by Ganser to have an organic basis and clouding of consciousness was observed in all his cases. Characteristics are approximate answers: incorrect but suggesting that the patient knows really; disorientation; hallucinations; short duration, with abrupt recovery and complete amnesia for the episode. This is a RARE condition, precipitated by emotional trauma and brief physical illness. It is essentially hysterical.

Hysterical infantilism: regression is a common hysterical response to stress, encouraged in physical illness. The invalid is put to bed and cared for like a child. In a severe hysterical reaction to stress or conflict the patient may act out a desire to return to infancy and talk or cry like a baby, eat with his fingers, wet himself and crawl instead of walk. A woman of 40, mildly spastic, with few resources developed infantilism when her mother died.

Hysterical psychosis: this consists of grossly disturbed behaviour coming on with dramatic suddenness, apparently in reaction to an upsetting event, and manifest in hallucinations (visual and auditory), delusions, screaming and bizarre activity. It seldom lasts more than a matter of days, but sedation with chlorpromazine in 100 mg doses may be needed during this period.

BRIQUET'S SYNDROME (SOMATIZATION DISORDER)

-   affects women of under 35 at its onset.
-   multiple symptoms, including gynaecological and sexual, not all necessarily of the conversion type.
-   numerous contacts with different doctors and hospitals.
-   histrionic personality.
-   long course - 20-30 years - ranging over various systems.

67

- dysharmony in relationships, marital and with children.
- genetic link: 20% female relatives have similar problems, and male relatives tend to antisocial personality.

Complications
- repeated surgery, some unnecessary
- dependence on prescribed drugs
- parasuicide
- divorce

Hypochondriasis: this is closely related to Briquet's syndrome but also affects men. The patient is preoccupied with the fear of physical or mental disease and constantly finds "proof" of its presence in his normal bodily functions and appearance, or the most trivial deviations. There is not usually such a variety of symptoms as in Briquet but a similar strain is put upon family and professionals.

MANAGEMENT OF HYSTERICAL PATIENTS

Since hysterical patients of all types have a particular aversion to psychiatrists and change their hospital doctors and surgeons as casually as clothes, it usually falls to the lot of the primary care physician to treat them.

Patience, realism and **sound medical acumen** are essentials. To avoid **polypharmacy** and/or **multiple investigations**, reinforcers of hysterical symptomatology, the doctor needs to feel secure in his diagnosis: by remaining particularly clinically alert with these patients, looking for **objective signs** of disease, and making physical examinations as necessary.

Psychiatric illness: hysterical symptoms may arise secondarily to any disease, particularly depression (see also Chapter 5). Evidence of depression includes impaired sleep, appetite, energy, interests, low mood, weight loss, hopelessness. In a minority of cases clinical depression will require medication, usually most successfully an MAOI such as phenelzine 45-60 mg daily: with careful instructions about dietary and other precautions.

Medication: apart from the situation above **its place is severely limited, despite pressure to prescribe** hypnotics, diuretics, analgesics, anti-inflammatory drugs, anti-spasmodics, antibiotics, and - especially - anxiolytics. Tricyclic antidepressants and phenothiazines produce severe side effects in these patients.

Relaxation techniques should be learned from a physiotherapist or in a lay class, and commercial audiotapes help the patient to relax and to sleep.
Exceptionally, with major conversion symptoms, dramatic treatment is the most likely to persuade the patient to relinquish her

stance: a course of 3 slow, intravenous injections of diazepam (10-20 mg) combined with suggestion allows the patient a dignified exit from, say, paralysis, with the feeling that the doctor has taken the suffering seriously.

Hypnosis theoretically serves a similar purpose, and hysterical patients usually make good subjects. Dangers are of inducing undue personal dependence, or that to please the doctor the patient will feign a trance and fail to benefit.

The therapeutic alliance with the patient is the keystone of useful treatment. It must include mutual respect, and on the doctor's side an appreciation of the patient's deep emotional difficulties. Hysterical patients, for all their apparent superficiality and importunate demands are profoundly disappointed with themselves and feel helpless. These feelings stem from unsatisfactory relationships with both parents in early life, which colour and distort all other relationships and the patients' own self-image. The goal is final self-acceptance through emotional maturity.

Behavioural principles underpin and strengthen the support and encouragement offered to the patient during discussions. Offer a preset course of 3-6 sessions to work on current problems, not to be reduced with recovery or extended without. Failure and complaints are dealt with summarily; achievement brings the rewards of interest and praise. Small tasks are set to make achievement easy: contacting an old friend, taking a walk, work. Insist that every day the patient does one thing purely for herself: buying some flowers, listening to music....

Family involvement: often family and friends are the chief collaborators in insisting that the patient is physically ill, and reinforce her symptoms. If they can be helped to understand the situation and also reward the patient for being well rather than ill, recovery will be easier. Often, however, the patient's mother or other relative has a similar personality and relishes the drama of sickness and is bored with health.

MANAGEMENT OF PATIENTS WITH PERSISTENT PSYCHOGENIC PAIN

There is every reason for emotional conflicts and stresses to be converted through hysterical mechanisms into pain: often symbolically sited. A lonely widow felt aching in the vagina, a worried student had headaches. Persistent head, back, abdominal or pelvic pain that has been exhaustively investigated should be regarded as substantially psychogenic and treated accordingly:

- a finite number of discussion sessions (up to 10 in pain patients)
- gradual withdrawal from analgesics and anxiolytics: with praise

for the smallest success.
- teaching in relaxation.
- similar achievement and reward techniques during psychotherapy as described above.

NEVER suggest that pain is imagined.

CHILDREN AND HYSTERIA

An adult with a hysterical personality is often denigrated as "immature". This does not mean she is like a normal child. A youngster displaying the same egocentricity and attention-seeking would be called "spoiled". Children of all ages but most obviously from about 8 years upwards can suffer various hysterical symptoms:

- histrionic personality with tantrums,
- enuresis, encopresis,
- nervous cough,
- aphonia,
- abdominal and other pains, nausea and vomiting,
- infantilism - usually to the stage of a feared rival: a new sibling,
- fantastic lying.

The underlying dynamics are similar to those for adults: conflicting feelings about a key figure: say an incestuous father, or a mother neurotically or physically ill; examinations and the feared response of an autocratic father to failure; depressed, unemployed or otherwise inauthentic father; divorce or threats of separation; sexual dysharmony between the parents. Escape from school or other responsibility can induce symptoms in a child as in an adult. Management: this involves couples therapy for the parents, if together, family therapy including the child, and individual sessions to support him. Since this is time-consuming referral to a Child Guidance Clinic may be prudent.

EPIDEMIC HYSTERIA

Common characteristics:

- often in a school or similar institution for the young
- predominantly females affected
- charismatic or prestigious person is first or early victim
- underlying state of transition or insecurity calling for a demonstration of cohesiveness in the community
- triggering factor may be a physical illness or event: a schoolgirl becoming pregnant, someone having a fit
- benign, self-limiting course, from a day to several months

It may remain endemic among vulnerable individuals, subject to hysterical disorders. Almost any symptoms may be involved but fainting is common, and in benign encephalomyelitis pains all over, weakness, loss of concentration, headache, irritability, menstrual disturbances have all been included.

Management

- awareness of the possibility
- break up the group of affected people
- avoid coercion or confrontation - these always fail
- provide clear information to all concerned
- treat patients as individuals, separately.

The culture-bound syndromes of latah, koro and amok may break out in epidemic form in Africa, or individually in the West. Motor symptoms and seemingly psychotic excitement predominate.

MUNCHAUSEN'S SYNDROME AND OTHER MALINGERING

Malingering, unlike hysteria, means the **conscious** production of symptoms or signs to **pretend illness.** There is understandable gain, often financial, and malingering may follow on a hysterical disorder that has attracted secondary gain.

Munchausen's syndrome occurs more often in men and is associated with severe personality problems. Such patients have long since lost all contact with relatives or friends. There seems to be a compulsive desire to get into a hospital and such manoeuvres as swallowing razor blades (often wrapped in plastic), infecting surgical wounds with faeces, or poking wire up the urethra to induce haematuria are commonplace. These patients begin by being plausible and pathetic, but discharge themselves in a rage if psychiatric help is offered. They are less likely to present at general practitioners' surgeries since they crave instant drama. Hysteria has no overlap with Munchausen, but that hysterical patients also like to be treated as physically ill.

REFERENCES

Fenton, G.W. (1986) Epilepsy and hysteria. British Journal of Psychiatry, **149**, 28-37
Lishman, W.A. (1978) Organic Psychiatry, Blackwell, Oxford
Roberts, J.K.A. (1984) Differential Diagnosis in Neuropsychiatry, Wiley, Chichester
Roy, A. (ed.) (1982) Hysteria, Wiley, Chichester
Thorley, A. (1986) Hysterical syndromes. In Hill, P., Murray, R., Thorley, A. (eds.) Essentials of Postgraduate Psychiatry II, Grune and Stratton, London
Trimble, M.R. (1981) Neuropsychiatry, Wiley, Chichester

8

Frightened patients

Maurice Lipsedge

QUICK REFERENCE GUIDE

SORTING PROCESS: A DIFFERENTIAL DIAGNOSIS OF FEAR

1. Is there fluctuating clouding of consciousness, inattention and disorientation? Look for an **acute organic basis** - e.g. drug intoxication or withdrawal, infective, metabolic or endocrine cause etc.
2. Is the patient being frightened by delusions of persecution or hallucinations in clear consciousness? Look for other features of **schizophrenia, affective psychosis or paranoid state.**
3. Does the patient irrationally avoid certain objects or situations, or have difficulty leaving home unaccompanied? The probable

diagnosis is phobic anxiety state, including agoraphobia and social problems.

4. Does the patient experience recurrent panic attacks? Think of **panic disorder**. Exclude benzodiazepine and alcohol dependence and other organic causes.

5. Does the patient have obsessional ruminations or rituals? If so, the diagnosis is likely to be **obsessional neurosis**. Look for a primary depressive illness.

6. Does the patient have generalised anxiety and tension and autonomic hyperactivity, with no obvious immediate precipitants? The diagnosis is likely to be **anxiety state** - exclude thyrotoxicosis.

7. Does the patient have recurrent re-experiencing of traumatic events? The diagnosis is likely to be **post-traumatic stress disorder**.

FEAR AND ANXIETY AS A REACTION TO PHYSICAL ILLNESS OR ITS TREATMENT

Doctors will frequently encounter fear, apprehension and anxiety as understandable reactions to physical illness or its treatment. Fear can be induced by threatened loss, such as possible impairment of working capacity, or sexual potency, and by life threatening illnesses, such as myocardial infarction or malignancy. Referral for investigation, or admission to hospital itself, can obviously generate anxiety as well, especially the sight of seriously ill or dying patients, and the alarming presence of complicated and impersonal technical apparatus, electronic monitors and infusion lines. People with certain personality configurations are particularly prone to develop anxiety states when confronted with physical illness, especially for the first time. This group will include physical fitness enthusiasts and patients with anxious or obsessional predispositions, who find it difficult to tolerate uncertainty. Fear and anxiety in physically ill patients and their relatives can be reduced by giving them careful and unhurried explanations of the nature of the physical illness, the significance of the symptoms, the reasons for investigations, the aim of treatment, and the probable outcome.

PROTRACTED TERMINAL ILLNESS

Patients with protracted terminal illnesses may become frightened and their anxiety may show itself as demanding or irritable behaviour. Dying patients often fear physical distress, disfigurement, or uncontrollable pain, as well as loss of personal dignity due to incontinence and helplessness. They might also be afraid of being abandoned by their families, or even by nursing or medical staff. Other patients with terminal illnesses may use the psychological defence mechanism of denial to protect themselves against distress, and they may appear to be unaware of the gravity of their condition, having suppressed intolerable fear. Clinicians must be sensitive to this state to avoid major problems in communication. Patients must be given the opportunity to ventilate distress and fear, and to talk about their grief over impending losses. They must be reassured that their pain will be relieved.

ANXIETY DISORDERS

Between two and four per cent of the population suffers at some time from a disorder in which fear or anxiety, are the main presenting symptoms. The most practical way to approach the frightened patient is to determine whether the fear is persistent and pervasive, or whether it occurs in waves of panic.

The term **GENERALISED ANXIETY STATE** refers to a more or less continuous **condition of diffuse, pervasive fear and apprehension, accompanied by physical symptoms**. Generalised anxiety is sometimes referred to as "free-floating anxiety". Physical sensations include muscle tension and unpleasant feelings associated with overactivity of the autonomic nervous system, including **palpitations, sweating, shakiness and diarrhoea. Sleep is shallow**, interrupted and unrefreshing. There may be **tension headaches and hyperventilation**. Other autonomic accompaniments of anxiety **include dry mouth and "butterfly" feelings** in the stomach.

Nearly thirty per cent of psychiatric consultations in general practice are by patients with generalised anxiety states, with **women** being affected **more often than men**. The onset generally occurs in early adult life. There tends to be a positive family history of anxiety states, and questioning about childhood might reveal "separation anxiety". Enquiries should be directed at uncovering recent or current conflict, such as opposing responsibilities (e.g. duty to family versus loyalty to an employer), or excessive stress. The possibility that the anxiety symptoms are based on an underlying depressive illness should be borne in mind, and the patient should be questioned about the presence of early morning waking, diurnal variation in mood, and ideas of guilt, remorse, pessimism and suicide. Poor concentration and impaired appetite and weight loss can, of course, occur in both anxiety and depression. Furthermore, **it is not uncommon for depressive neuroses and anxiety states to co-exist**.

The term **PANIC DISORDER** refers to recurrent attacks of anxiety that can occur at any time but may be more likely to happen in certain situations, especially crowded and enclosed places. The patient will report **bouts of intense fear and apprehension**, sometimes with a **sensation of imminent disaster or death**, accompanied by feelings of **unreality**.

Physical concomitants include **palpitations, difficulty in breathing and swallowing, weakness of the legs, sweating and faintness, and hyperventilation** commonly occurs. By reducing the level of carbon dioxide in the blood, overbreathing decreases cerebral blood flow by up to forty per cent. **Hyperventilation** may cause paraesthesia in the hands and feet, and around the mouth, and, if severe, carpopedal muscle spasms of the hands or "main d'accoucheur", due to tetany caused by alkalosis. Other associated physical symptoms include blurring of vision and muscle cramps. The symptoms produced by hyperventilation may be confined to one side of the body and might suggest the presence of a focal intracranial lesion. The distinction between focal cerebral disease, causing unilateral somatic symptoms and hyperventilation can be made by getting the patient to over-breathe. If voluntary hyperventilation reproduces symptoms then intracranial pathology is much less likely.

TREATMENT of anxiety states includes **reassurance and counselling**. A **thorough physical examination** will help allay the fear of a heart attack which so often accompanies panic attacks. It is helpful to explain to the patient how the autonomic nervous system functions and its adaptive role in "fight or flight" situations. Counselling sessions should be aimed at **eliciting specific cues which trigger off anxiety**, and at working out **coping strategies** which might help lessen the anxiety. Patients should be encouraged to confront rather than avoid fear-provoking situations. Anxiety states generally arise as a result of external stress acting on a susceptible personality but, in some cases, there is no discernable precipitant, and the patient's previous personality shows no anxiety trait. Questions should be asked about reliance on alcohol to suppress anxiety, as this is a maladaptive coping mechanism which can lead to alcohol dependence.

Psychotherapy might be indicated and the patient might benefit from marital or family therapy.

SPECIFIC TRAINING IN ANXIETY MANAGEMENT includes instruction in techniques of controlled breathing by Physiotherapists or Occupational Therapists, which can significantly reduce hyperventilation. Training in muscle relaxation is also very useful.

DRUG TREATMENT includes the use of benzodiazepines, which must only be given for a short period of time. The longer-acting benzodiazepines, such as diazepam, clorazepate, or clobazam, are less addictive than the short-acting minor tranquillizers, such as lorazepam or oxazepam. Clobazam has the added advantage of relatively little sedative effect. Beta-blockers are useful where anxiety is accompanied by distressing palpitations and tremor. Atenolol, 25-50 mg daily, and nadolol, 40 mg daily, are preferable to propranolol because they are less fat soluble and are, therefore, less likely to penetrate the brain and cause insomnia, nightmares and depression. Certain occupational groups, such as professional musicians, whose performance-anxiety leads to an incapacitating tremor of hands or lips, can benefit greatly from a beta-blocker taken on the day of a major concert or recording session. It is important to calibrate the dose against the therapeutic effect, and the patient should be advised to experiment with the drug before an actual performance. In those patients in whom anxiety and depression coexist, a sedative tricyclic antidepressant, such as amitriptyline, in a dose of 75-150 mg at night should be given.

The **PROGNOSIS OF ANXIETY STATES** clearly depends on the previous personality of the patient, with well-adjusted people making a more rapid and complete recovery. The complications of anxiety states include agoraphobia (see below) alcohol and tranquillizer dependence, and depression. It is important to bear in mind that anxiety may be a prodromal symptom of a depressive illness. The following conditions must be excluded: thyrotoxicosis, phaeochromocytoma, tranquillizer abuse and illicit drug abuse (see below).

PHOBIC DISORDERS

Phobic disorders are characterised by intense, irrational and uncontrollable fear of specific situations, activities, objects or creatures. (The word "phobia" is derived from the Greek word for terror or fear.) The phobia is disproportionate to any real danger inherent in the situation, and it leads to avoidance of the dreaded activity or situation, with a significant degree of suffering and impairment of daily life. The patient recognises that the fear is excessive and unreasonable.

Phobic disorders are conveniently divided into four separate states:

1. Agoraphobia
2. Social phobias
3. Animal phobias
4. Miscellaneous specific phobias.

Agoraphobia

Agoraphobia is the commonest of the severe phobic states. The majority of agoraphobic patients are women and symptoms usually start between the mid-teens and the mid-thirties. Although the term agoraphobia refers to an open space the disorder usually involves not only a morbid fear of going out alone, but also a fear of crowded and enclosed spaces, and especially supermarkets and public transport. Agoraphobics may also be intensely afraid of being alone at home, or in any public place from which escape may be difficult. They often feel reassured if they are accompanied by a relative or friend, or even by a shopping basket on wheels. Agoraphobia is often accompanied by free-floating anxiety, panic attacks and depersonalisation and derealisation (see below). The patient is afraid of having a panic attack (anticipatory fear) and becomes reluctant to enter a variety of situations associated with panic attacks. Depression commonly occurs in agoraphobia, both as a reaction to the disability, and as a mood disturbance which might have been present from the onset of the phobic anxiety state. Questioning of relatives often reveals an anxious and dependent premorbid personality, with a history of childhood fears and separation

76

anxiety. The disorder might be precipitated by major life events or conflicts in relationships with husband, mother or adult children. The disorder may persist for many years, giving rise to the "housebound housewife syndrome". Although ostensibly a very handicapping disorder, agoraphobia may confer a degree of manipulative power on the sufferer, as in the case of a jealous wife who controls her husband's movements by requiring him to telephone her at home every hour to reassure her when she is alone. Agoraphobics may come to rely on alcohol and tranquillizers to relieve their anxiety and might develop chemical dependence.

Social phobias

These states are characterised by a persistent and irrational fear of situations in which the individual might be exposed to scrutiny by other people, or a fear that the sufferer will inadvertantly react in a way which might evoke shame or embarrassment, such as vomiting in public, or even blushing. The patient might also have a morbid fear of shaking or choking in interpersonal situations. This leads to an avoidance of social situations and may end in severe reclusiveness. There might be other psychiatric disorders associated with social phobias, such as depression or paranoid personality. Social phobias are much less common than agoraphobia and, unlike agoraphobia, are only slightly more common in women than men. Social phobias can lead to occupational impairment, as in the clerk who is afraid that his hand might shake when writing in public. Social life in such patients is restricted by fear of uncontrollably rattling a teacup on its saucer, or a dread of making a noise when eating in public, or appearing tremulous when addressing a meeting.

Animal phobias

These consist of an intense fear of small animals, with onset in childhood. Generally the personality in animal phobias is much less impaired than people with agoraphobia, or even social phobias. At times however the phobia can severely restrict daily life, as in a young mother whose morbid fear of feathers prevented her going into the garden.

Miscellaneous specific phobias include intense irrational fears of thunderstorms, heights and darkness. Thunder phobics repeatedly telephone the Meteorological Office for reassurance that a storm is not approaching, while fears of heights and of darkness can lead to obvious impairment of routine activities. Flying phobics may have a panic attack at the prospect of boarding a plane, or as the plane is about to take off or land.

School phobia, or school refusal, presents as a severe anxiety focussed on entering the school premises in schoolchildren of any age, often with somatization of anxiety, which then presents as nausea, vomiting, diarrhoea or abdominal pains occurring just before it is time to leave home for school. Although the child might appear moody and irritable, he is not anxious when separated from his mother outside the school situation. Thus, he might be able to go to the shops by himself, without showing any undue fear or anxiety. School phobia is not a homogeneous disorder and there may be a variety of underlying problems, including bullying or academic difficulties, or marital discord in the parents. About one fifth of the mothers of school phobic adolescents suffer from psychiatric disorder. In some cases, the mother of a school-refusing child will be found to be suffering from a fear of being alone, and to be covertly encouraging her child to stay at home.

Treatment of phobias

Treatment consists of behaviour therapy, either alone, or in a combination with drug therapy. The behavioural therapy of phobias has three components:

1. Systematic desensitisation.
2. Prolonged exposure.
3. Modelling.

In **SYSTEMATIC DESENSITISATION** the patient is gradually exposed to the phobic stimulus up a hierarchy of increasing fearfulness. The exposure is paired with relaxation training and takes place first in fantasy and then in real life situations until the patient habituates to the stimulus. The more specific phobias respond best to this approach.

PROLONGED EXPOSURE: This takes place first in imagination and then "in vivo" with maximum exposure to the feared stimulus or situation, until habituation occurs. This technique is especially valuable in patients with a significant degree of free-floating anxiety.

MODELLING: The patient is required to observe and then imitate the therapist handling or exposing himself to the feared stimulus.

Agoraphobia is generally regarded as the most resistant of the phobias and it responds best to a combination of modelling and prolonged exposure under cover of waning doses of a benzodiazepine, such as diazepam, supplemented if necessary by a beta-blocker.

Drug treatment of phobics

Antidepressants, both tricyclic (such as clomipramine), and monoamine-oxidase inhibitors (MAOIs) might be helpful adjuncts to behaviour therapy in the management of agoraphobia. Of the MAOIs, phenelzine is more effective than isocarboxazid and safer than tranylcypramine. It should be given in doses of up to 75-90 mg daily. The patient must be warned to avoid tyramine containing food-stuffs (cheese, yeast, meat extracts and fermented forms of alcohol and beverages) and drugs containing pressor agents (such as ephedrine) and most of the tricyclic antidepressants.

While the MAOIs can certainly be effective, it is wiser to start with the less hazardous and addictive tricyclic antidepressants. If patients fail to improve with the tricyclic, it is important to allow a two week "wash out" period before switching from a tricyclic to an MAOI.

DEPERSONALISATION AND DEREALISATION

These often accompany phobic anxiety, especially agoraphobia, and involve unpleasant and frightening feelings that one's body and/or the outside world has changed. The terms refer to an alteration in the individual's perception of his body image, with a feeling of strangeness, detachment and unreality, in relation to himself and to his immediate environment. The patient feels like an automaton, and feels as if he is observing his own behaviour from outside. Other people appear like robots or puppets. The total experience of depersonalisation and derealisation is distinguished from a delusional state by the patient's awareness that his body and the world have **not really** changed - i.e. there is an "as if" quality to the entire experience. There might be other distortions or perceptions, deja vu and hallucinatory experiences, and the individual feels that he has lost his capacity to respond with emotional resonance to other people or to events. The distinction of depersonalisation and derealisation from temporal lobe epilepsy is dealt with below. Depersonalisation and derealisation commonly occur in phobic anxiety states but they are also found in a wide variety of other conditions, including fatigue, severe depression, schizophrenia, hypomania and alcohol, barbiturate and hallucinogen abuse, in addition to delirium (see below), temporal-parietal disease, and post head injury states.

HYPOCHONDRIASIS

This is an irrational fear of a serious illness, such as AIDS, heart disease or cancer, often based on a misinterpretation of normal bodily sensations. The fear of illness leads to a persistent but futile quest for medical reassurance. Hypochondriasis may be part of a depressive illness, while bizarre beliefs about the transformation of internal organs may occur in schizophrenia. There may be a fear of parasitic infection (Ekbom's syndrome). Where hypochondriasis is part of an endogenous depressive illness, then a tricyclic antidepressant or even electro-convulsive therapy, are indicated. So-called mono-symptomatic delusional hypochondriasis might respond to pimozide.

PARANOID STATES

Fear might be part of a paranoid state where the patient believes that he is the victim of persecution and that other people or organisations are trying to harm him, poison him, drive him insane or damage him in some other way. Paranoid states may develop in people with paranoid personalities - i.e persons who are hypersensitive and prone to misinterpret other people's behaviour as rejecting, critical or hostile. Paranoid ideas are particularly common among the deaf. Paranoid symptoms can also occur in association with a primary mental illness, such as schizophrenia, depression, hypomania or an organic psychiatric disorder, or they can be part of a discrete paranoid state, which is defined as a fixed delusional condition without prominent hallucinations.

OBSESSIONAL NEUROSIS

The symptoms of this disorder consist of **ruminations** and **rituals**. Ruminations are recurrent intrusive ideas or impulses which the patient finds frightening, repugnant, or offensive, but which he is unable to suppress. The thoughts might be obscene, violent or blasphemous and induce a state of tension.

Obsessional rituals are compulsive repetitive acts, such as cleaning or checking, which the patient feels obliged to perform because of an intense and irrational fear of contamination or violence. When the individual attempts to resist the compulsive urge to carry out a ritual, there is a sense of mounting tension that can generally be relieved by yielding to the compulsion.

Obsessional neurosis is equally common in men and women and generally begins in early adult life, often in people with perfectionist rigid personalities. Obsessional symptoms are also commonly found in depressive illnesses, and more rarely they can occur in schizophrenic and organic brain syndromes. The treatment of **obsessional neurosis** includes both chemotherapy and behaviour therapy. Any underlying depressive illness should be treated with an antidepressant and clomipramine is claimed to be particularly useful for this disorder, whilst trazodone might also be effective. If tricyclic antidepressants fail, then a trial of ECT should be considered. If all other methods fail, then psycho-surgery might be the last resort.

Obsessional rituals can be treated by a combination of **prolonged exposure, modelling**, and **response prevention**. The therapist may carry out these procedures in the patient's own home, where the patient is encouraged to have contact with objects which he regards as contaminating. The therapist also touches the contaminants and then supervises the patient and distracts or diverts him from carrying out washing or checking rituals. Ruminations are less amenable to behaviour therapy but might respond to procedures such as satiation or thought-stopping.

POST-TRAUMATIC STRESS DISORDER

There may be a history of a psychologically traumatic event, such as assault, rape, an accident, or a natural disaster, which produces anxiety together with a characteristic cluster of symptoms. These include recurrent or intrusive recollections of the event, frequent dreams of the trauma, and suddenly acting or feeling as if the traumatic event were recurring, triggered off by a chance association. This condition, known as post-traumatic stress disorder, might be accompanied by a feeling of detachment or estrangement ("psychic numbing"), as well as impairment of concentration, insomnia and phobic avoidance of activities which recall the original traumatic event. This disorder is best treated by a combination of psychotherapy, behaviour therapy for any phobic avoidance, and an antidepressant if there is a significant depressive component.

THE FRIGHTENED PATIENT AND EPILEPSY

Emotional disturbances can result from a discharging lesion in the temporal lobe and episodic attacks of anxiety must be distinguished from temporal lobe epilepsy, especially as the most common emotion associated with epilepsy is fear. The differentiation is particularly difficult when there are sudden panic attacks accompanied by marked depersonalisation, since both might be accompanied by deja vu and distortions of perception and, rarely, patients with severe anxiety states might also report hallucinations. There have been reports of patients with severe anxiety states fainting when their anxiety is at its most intense level, thus making the distinction from epilepsy even harder. Differentiation between the two conditions lies in the fact that anxiety symptoms will persist between episodes in patients with neurosis, and the episodes might have a more clearly obvious emotional trigger. Episodes both begin and terminate abruptly in temporal lobe epilepsy, but although they may start suddenly in anxious patients, they tend to end much more gradually than in epileptics, in whom there is a relatively rapid resolution. The epileptics also have a characteristic "march" in the evolution of their symptoms and some degree of alteration of consciousness is a major feature, while consciousness remains clear in anxiety states. Epileptics also have disturbances of speech and show automatic behaviour which neurotic patients do not, and in temporal lobe epilepsy the fear is often accompanied by visceral sensory symptoms, including epigastric discomfort, flushing, sweating and palpitations. Epileptic phenomena tend to have a stereotyped quality. Neurotic patients tend to have evidence of over-dependence in their histories, and a family history of neurosis, while the patient with temporal lobe disorders might have a history of disease leading to cerebral damage (severe birth trauma, prolonged anoxia, head injury with loss of consciousness, or infection: meningitis, encephalitis and mastoiditis). An EEG might help to confirm the diagnosis, but patients with epilepsy, especially temporal lobe epilepsy,

81

do have a raised incidence of neurotic symptoms, especially anxiety, quite apart from the phenomena associated with their seizures.

FEAR AS THE PRESENTING SYMPTOM OF AN ORGANIC DISORDER

The following organic disorders might present with symptoms of fear and anxiety:

1. Hyperthyroidism
2. Phaeochromocytoma
3. Hypocalcaemia
4. Insulinoma
5. Caffeinism
6. Benzodiazepine dependence
7. Acute organic brain disorders.

Hyperthyroidism

In addition to anxiety, the patient may have other psychological symptoms, including irritability and restlessness. The patient should be asked about temperature preference and weight loss despite increased appetite. On examination, there might be a goitre, a sleeping pulse greater than 90 per minute, tremor and atrial fibrillation. The diagnosis is confirmed by measurement of serum thyroxine.

Hypoparathyroidism

Patients with idiopathic or surgically-induced hypoparathyroidism, might present with nervousness and irritability. Other features of the disorder include tetany, cataracts and epilepsy and a low fasting calcium will confirm the diagnosis.

Phaeochromocytoma

Tumours of the adrenal medulla secrete adrenaline and nordrenaline. Secretion of these pressor agents can be continuous or paroxysmal, and can lead to intense anxiety, accompanied by palpitations, headache, pallor, sweating and shaking. The patient will generally be hypertensive between attacks and the diagnosis is confirmed by the presence of excessive amounts of catecholamines and their metabolites in the urine.

Insulinomas

These tumours cause bouts of hypoglycaemia, which are characterised by irritability and disinhibition and, at times, marked anxiety. The diagnosis is made by a low blood sugar and elevated serum insulin.

Caffeinism

Caffeine is a mild psychostimulant with sympathomimetic properties. When taken in excessive quantities (i.e. more than about 750 mg of caffeine per day), it can cause symptoms which can closely mimic an anxiety state. It has been observed that many heavy tranquillizer users also have a high caffeine intake. Caffeine is a competitive inhibitor of diazepam binding at the brain benzodiazepine receptor sites, and it has been suggested that people who chronically use benzodiazepines are, in fact, suffering from caffeinism, and anxiety symptoms which emerge on discontinuation of the benzodiazepine are caused by the anxiety-mimicking effect of the caffeine.

Benzodiazepine dependency syndromes

If diazepam, chlordiazepoxide, and other benzodiazepines are taken for a month in dosages two or three times the maximum recommended daily therapeutic dose, withdrawal symptoms of the barbiturate type occur when the benzodiazepine is abruptly stopped. Minor withdrawal symptoms consist of anxiety, insomnia, tremor and nightmares, while the major withdrawal syndrome includes all these symptoms together with grand mal seizures, psychosis and hyperpyrexia. Recently, physicians have become aware of **low dose dependency** on benzodiazepines in which signs and symptoms develop after a patient abruptly stops the long-term use of therapeutically prescribed doses of benzodiazepines. Symptoms attributed to therapeutic dose benzodiazepine withdrawal include anxiety, tension, agitation, breathlessness, irritability, tremor, nausea, insomnia, panic attacks, impairment of memory and concentration, perceptual alterations (hyperacusis, hypersensitivity to touch and pain), paraesthesia, feelings of unreality, visual hallucinations and tachycardia. Some of these symptoms may continue for weeks or even months, but tend to improve with time. Physiological signs associated with low dose benzodiazepine withdrawal include dilated pupils, increased pulse rate and increased blood pressure.

ACUTE ORGANIC PSYCHIATRIC SYNDROMES

Delirium, which is the term for any acute organic brain disorder, is characterised by impaired consciousness, diminished attention, disorientation and poor memory, plus disturbances of perception and orientation. The mood in delirium will range from anxiety to terror, and the patient may also be perplexed, hostile or suspicious, and, at times, might swing into apathy. Accompanying features include fatigue, restlessness, inability to think clearly, and vivid dreams and nightmares. The condition might progress to include illusions, hallucinations, delusions, distractability and overactivity. Familiar people are mis-identified and the patient may confabulate. There is typically a diurnal variation with relatively clear consciousness in the morning and increasing fear as the night approaches. There may be reversal of the sleep-wakefulness cycle, with daytime drowsiness and severe insomnia.

Causes of delirium include alcohol and other toxins - e.g. heavy metals, cerebrovascular, heart and pulmonary disease, collagenosis, endocrine and metabolic disorders, cerebral tumours and infections (encephalitis, meningitis, and abscess), epilepsy, head injury and post-operative states.

In addition to the hallucinogens (see below) they include anti-cholinergic drugs, steroids, L-dopa, anti-convulsants, anti-histamines, cimetedine, and barbiturates. Finally, acute organic reactions can be caused by lack of vitamins, including thiamine, nicotinic acid, B_{12} and folic acid.

In acute organic reactions, the first priority is to establish the underlying physical disorder. The psychiatric differential diagnosis is based on the history of a recent and acute onset of disturbed behaviour, and physical illness, together with disorientation or other evidence of impaired consciousness, which do not occur in anxiety states or the functional psychoses.

FEAR AND CHEMICAL DEPENDENCE

Fear, amounting to terror, might be encountered in acute **alcohol withdrawal states**. In the milder withdrawal states, anxiety and apprehension, especially in the morning, might be accompanied by tremor, sweating, nausea and "heaves". In full-blown delirium tremens, which can occur two to seven days after withdrawal of alcohol, there are profound confusion, vivid hallucinations, which are mainly visual, delusions and intense fear, insomnia, restlessness, with progression to agitation, together with disorientation and marked tremulousness and slurring of speech. There are signs of autonomic nervous system overactivity, with dilated pupils, tachycardia, fever and sweating. Convulsions can occur in over ten per cent of patients with delirium tremens, and a similar picture is seen in abrupt withdrawal from barbiturates and benzodiazepines (see above). Management includes careful nursing in a well-lit, quiet room, and a systematic search for associated injury or infection, especially cerebral laceration, subdural haematoma, pneumonia and meningitis. Specific treatment includes rehydration, high potency intravenous parentrovite, carbamazepine and chlormethiazole, together with an antibiotic if there is an intercurrent infection.

84

ALCOHOLIC HALLUCINOSIS

This can occur without the features of delirium tremens - i.e. with no clouding of consciousness, and is characterised by threatening and hostile voices. There may also be unstructured sounds, such as clicking, buzzing or ringing. One patient was so convinced of the reality of these threatening voices that he requested help from the police. After being sent away from the police station, his menacing voices persisted and he deliberately broke the window of a neighbouring jewellers shop in order to be arrested and taken into protective custody.

The hallucinated voices might discuss the patient or address him directly, and they tend to develop in the first twenty-four to forty-eight hours after the complete cessation of drinking in an alcoholic, and generally subside within a week, although, in a small proportion of patients, hallucinations can become chronic.

ILLICIT DRUGS

Cocaine is increasingly encountered as a drug of abuse. It is taken by sniffing, smoking or injection, and can cause paranoid psychosis and tactile hallucinations (formication). On examination, there is evidence of sympathetic overactivity with tachycardia and dilated pupils.

Amphetamines: When used chronically, and taken orally or intravenously, amphetamines can also induce anxiety and paranoid ideas with auditory, visual or tactile hallucinations. Again there is evidence of sympathetic hyperstimulation, with tachycardia, dilated pupils and hyperreflexia.

Lysergic acid diethylamide (LSD), mescaline and psylocybin (found in certain mushrooms in Britain): These hallucinogens are taken orally. Their acute effects occur after about thirty minutes and are associated with illusions and, occasionally, hallucinations. "A bad trip" consists of terrifying perceptual distortions and depersonalisation and derealisation, and there may be intense anxiety and fear of self-disintegration, leading to an acute panic attack. "Flash backs" occur for up to one year after ingestion, especially after prolonged use of hallucinogens. "Flash backs" consist of vivid visual images or perceptual distortions which are accompanied by fear amounting to panic.

Solvent abuse

The inhalation or sniffing of volatile solvents, including commercial and domestic products such as paint-thinners, glue and lacquer, which can contain volatile hydrocarbons such as toluene, benzene and acetone, is indulged in by teenagers or young adults, mainly males. There are sporadic outbreaks of glue sniffing among adolescents in a school or neighbourhood. Hydrocarbon inhalation is usually a group activity, although some inhalers progress from group to solitary sniffing. Solvent abuse can lead to perceptual distortions, delusions and fear, in addition to physical symptoms of dizziness, slurred speech and ataxia. The glue sniffer might have a characteristic rash, caused by the repeated application of a plastic bag to the nose.

Opiates

The abstinence syndrome associated with opiate (heroin and methadone) withdrawal develops within about twenty-four hours of the last dose of opiate, and includes anxiety, in addition to craving, yawning, lacrimation, running nose, sweating, muscle twitching, restlessness, diarrhoea and dilated pupils. With heroin withdrawal, these symptoms gradually subside after the second or third day, but methadone withdrawal symptoms generally only reach maximum intensity after several days. Clonidine is the most satisfactory drug for alleviating these symptoms (see also Chapter 18).

9

The presentation and care of the rape victim

Gillian C. Mezey

QUICK REFERENCE GUIDE

SUMMARY

As sexual assault, in common with other crimes of violence, becomes more frequent, it is inevitable that GP's, alongside other health professionals, will be looked to as, not only the first line but frequently the only source of support for the victim. Recognising the reactions of rape victims and maintaining a non-critical attitude are important first steps. Ultimately, the victim will need to be supported until she has regained a sense of control over her life and can be said to be, no longer a victim, but a survivor.

BACKGROUND

Forcible rape is defined as the subjection of a women to sexual intercourse, without her consent. (Sexual Amendment Act 1976). The majority of women do not report the crime. It is estimated that three to four rapes are committed for every one reported[1]. Reasons for the reluctance to report include the woman's fear that her claim will be met by scepticism by the police.

87

There is little help available for the non-reporting woman: hospitals lack the facilities or, as often, the expertise to provide help and are generally reluctant to get involved in case legal proceedures are to be instituted[2]. Most rape crisis centres adopt a "feminist" approach, which is not always welcomed or beneficial to the woman. A number of victims contact volunteer organisations such as the Samaritans, some approach the Church, some their friends or family and, inevitably, for a number of rape victims, the first person they talk to about the rape will be their GP.

Although sex is involved, rape is primarily an expression of violence and reflects a power inbalance between two individuals. Where such an inbalance exists, it is easily abused, leading to children becoming victims of incest and even men, particularly in an institutionalised setting, may be sexually assaulted[3].

In describing her experience, the rape victim will generally focus on her fear and humiliation and her total loss of control over the situation. The anger and frustration expressed through rape is often preceded by a variety of criminal acts of violence. Studies on incarcerated rapists confirm that many of them not only have other sexual partners[4], but also extensive criminal records of non-sexual violence[5].

The misconception of rape as essentially a sexual act is responsible for the damaging effects on the victim and the acute sense of shame and guilt she feels afterwards. There are common societal and cultural attitudes that the victim may have enjoyed the experience, that rape somehow gratifies women's masochistic fantasies, that force heightens the excitement for both partners and the paradox that nice girls don't say "yes" but that "no" should not be accepted as a true reflection of their wishes. These beliefs are uncommon in non-sexual violence, when the boundary between the innocent victim and guilty offender is more clearly defined. In rape, the victim and rapist are often depicted as conspirators in some perverse but mutually gratifying drama: the rape victim seen as a vengeful seductress with the law as the only protection for the wrongfully accused, innocent man[6].

Societal misconceptions about rape isolate and stigmatise the rape victim more than victims of other forms of crime. Rape victims will often pretend they have been mugged or assaulted rather than raped, fearing the critical attitude of friends, wishing to avoid the curiosity, anger or shock that the revelation of rape creates.

There is no typical rape victim profile. The victim stereotype of young, attractive, middle-class, white female being raped is, more often than not, a myth. The likelihood of a woman being raped are similar to her chances of being subjected to any form of victimisation, i.e. rape victims are mostly young adult women, but elderly women, young children and pregnant mothers are not immune to this crime.

The effects of rape on the victim have been described as the "rape trauma syndrome"[7] and closely resemble the reactions found in victims of other types of external crises. Traumatophobia or fear of trauma was described in the 1940s: symptoms of anxiety, hysteria, insomnia and decreased sexual libido occurring in soldiers following war combat[8]. Similar psychological reactions are found in victims of kidnappings and sieges[9], of community disaster[10], and muggings[11], suggesting that these apparently diverse events have a common basis i.e. they engender fear and at the same time are perceived by the victim as being outside his or her control.

THE RAPE TRAUMA SYNDROME (Table 1)

The rape trauma syndrome is a two-stage reaction, generally lasting from three to four months. The woman's distress may either be "expressed" or "controlled", when little overt distress is immediately evident. In the more common "expressed" presentation, the woman will show extreme anxiety, fear and distress, reflecting her inner state of chaos. Physical complaints and alterations in behaviour are also frequently present. For the majority, these symptoms begin to resolve after days to weeks and at three to four months the memory of the rape experience should have receded far enough back in conscious awareness to allow a resumption to a previous normal level of functioning[12]. A number of women have more difficulty in coming to terms with and reorganising their lives following a rape and develop severe atypical and persistent reactions. One of the determinants of

Table 1   THE RAPE TRAUMA SYNDROME

ACUTE PHASE: DISORGANISATION (days - weeks)	Somatic reactions	Physical trauma Skeletal muscle tension Gastrointestinal irritability Genitourinary disturbance
	Emotional reactions	Shame and self-disgust Specific phobias Tearfulness Generalised anxiety Guilt and self-blame
LONG-TERM PROCESS: REORGANISATION (weeks - months)	Behaviour	Moving residence Increasing dependence on others Altered social activity Altered sexual behaviour/ enjoyment
	Psychological	Nightmares and flashbacks Rape-related phobias Increased sense of vulnerability Alteration in self-concept/ self-esteem

this so-called "compound" reaction[13] is the woman's pre-rape adjustment: poor psychosocial functioning, previous victimisation, past psychiatric treatment, a history of drug or alcohol abuse prior to the rape all make subsequent problems more likely.

One question that inevitably arises in the course of counselling rape victims is "What did she do to stop the attack?" In law, rape depends on demonstrating that the woman did not consent to have sexual intercourse. Non-consent is difficult to prove especially since there are generally no witnesses present and therefore the amount of resistance put up by the woman or the presence of actual physical injuries is often taken as evidence of non-consent i.e. the woman's claim must be genuine. Similarly, submissive and passive behaviour during a rape is sometimes interpreted by the victim's friends, family, the police and jury members as evidence that she welcomed or even enjoyed the rape. The woman herself may find it very difficult to understand and explain her inability to act effectively during the rape, particularly if beforehand she had regarded herself as a strong assertive person. It should always be remembered, however, that the context in which her inaction occurs is a life-threatening one, turning learned rational responses into life preserving reflex behaviour[14]. For the majority of victims who do not fight back, submissive behaviour does have the effect of preventing further serious physical injury. However, in the absence of resistance, without any physical evidence of her violation, the woman may find that her claim is treated with scepticism.

Rape victims are frequently unable to express the anger and outrage that her family and society will show. The woman is not only unable to blame the rapist, but she will frequently present herself as the guilty party. The act of rape forces her into the most intimate of human contacts, normally associated with love, trust and mutuality, but which, in this case, is motivated by anger and hatred and a wish to humiliate. The woman may believe that since sexual intercourse has taken place, the rapist "loves" her: if he loves her, then she must have done something to create it, i.e. "I am responsible for the rape!" It is paradoxical that the very person who is threatening to kill her is the same person who has the power to set her free. Any small act of mercy by the rapist is interpreted as kindness, a sign of reprieve, giving the hope that perhaps he has begun to care for her and will free her. If this occurs i.e. he allows her to live, it may be this "saviour" quality that is retained afterwards by the victim. In this respect, rape resembles other terrorist situations, where the victims feel their lives to be in danger and a close identification, even very positive feelings may develop between victim and aggressor. The victim's profound guilt and self blame and her apparent lack of anger towards the rapist (some even find themselves thanking him after the ordeal), will seem incomprehensible, unless the peculiar nature of the rape experience is understood.

COUNSELLING THE RAPE VICTIM

The first stage in management is accurate assessment of the urgency of the situation. This is generally related to how recently the rape has taken place. In an "acute" case i.e. 24-48 hours previously, the first decision to be made is whether the woman wishes to report the rape to the police. It is important to encourage her to decide this herself: a common reaction to rape victims is to infantilise them, removing their control by making decisions for them, albeit "for their own good" and it is important to guard against this. In practice, the earlier a rape is reported to the police, the greater the chance there is of that report being believed and followed up, of the rapist being caught and a conviction being secured. The longer the delay, the smaller the chances of a successful outcome and the benefits of reporting after a delay of more than 48 hours are questionable.

If the victim chooses to report, further medical management should be left to the police surgeon as the physical examination and specimens taken will provide essential forensic evidence in court.

With the non-reporting case, there are three main lines of management:

1. Medical

a. Physical examination and treatment of any associated physical injury.
b. Post-coital contraception.
c. Prevention/treatment of venereal infection - may require referral to a special clinic.

Psychotropic medication is rarely indicated in the management of the woman's acute distress and should be avoided as far as possible.

2. Practical

a. Rehousing - may require a medical recommendation.
b. Compensation.
   The majority of rape victims do not receive compensation simply because of the lack of awareness that they are entitled to it[15] and they should be encouraged to contact the CICB (Criminal Injuries Compensation Board).
c. Referring on to other agencies.
   - Special clinics
   - Citizen's Advice Bureau
   - Women's Refuge
   - Victim Support Schemes
   - General Hospitals
   - CICB
   - Rape Crisis Centres

3. Psychological

The therapeutic model used in treating rape victims in the acute stage is crisis intervention[7]. The assumptions behind this model are:

a. One is dealing with an individual who has been normal prior to the rape.
b. The rape represents a crisis, external to the woman's control, precipitating her into a state of turmoil. Her preconceptions about herself, those around her and her environment are shattered. The sooner the intervention is initiated, the more successful that intervention will be in returning the woman to her previously normal self and in preventing "maladaptive" responses from developing, e.g. she may become housebound and agoraphobic or use alcohol or drugs to help her cope with the overwhelming anxiety.

The most important aspect of counselling a victim of rape is that of sympathetic and non-judgemental listening. She will be frightened of criticism and frequently will have no other person to whom she can speak freely about her ordeal. For the listener, this is not only time consuming but also requires emotional energy: the experiences described are invariably painful and shocking to hear and rarely leave the listener unaffected.

It is essential to break what many victims refer to as a conspiracy of silence surrounding them. The woman fears burdening her husband, children and friends with her distress. The husband may not mention it, either to protect her feelings or because he fears his own, unpredictable responses. The effects of this silence are two-fold: firstly it reinforces the woman's belief that what has happened to her is too shameful to talk about. Secondly, it allows the fantasies of those close to the victim to grow into proportions of terrifying and often unrealistic intensity, until it becomes impossible to talk about the rape. Allowing the victim to ventilate her feelings is similar to the concept of guided mourning used in bereavement counselling.

The efforts to protect the woman from distress may continue for long after the rape and she may gradually find herself giving up her independence and autonomy. One young woman described how, having returned to live with her parents following the rape, they started censoring the newspapers and television for anything violent or potentially upsetting, which they would protect her from. The tendancy to infantilise rape victims, perhaps created through the initial dependence on others following the rape, both reflects and perpetuates the helplessness she experiences during the rape.

In counselling the rape victim, it is important to recognise that she forms part of a social network whose responses to her as "rape victim" will be crucial in determining the course of her recovery. The members of the family closest to the victim will inevitably be deeply affected by what has happened and, in a sense, can be seen

as secondary victims. They are frequently left confused and excluded from the frenzy of activity and concern surrounding the
victim[16].

The family should be included in any counselling offered to the
victim. Without this involvement their own hurt and confusion may
lead them, in turn, to reject or blame the victim at a time when she
most needs their support.

Some consideration should be given to the woman's life stage in
focusing on what this attack means to this patient at this particular
time: for an adolescent girl, the rape will threaten her emerging
sexuality and create conflicts over her wish for independence and
the threat this now represents. The rape of a married woman may
lead her to question her role as a wife and mother ...." if I am unable to look after myself, how can I possibly trust myself to look
after the children?"[17].

Rape victims should not be considered psychiatrically ill by
virtue of their victimisation alone. The anguish, expressed initially,
is not necessarily "illness" but a crisis which, in the majority of
cases will resolve within a few months. In certain cases, who
develop the chronic compound reaction, psychiatric referral may be
appropriate.

Table 2 RELATIVE INDICATIONS FOR REFERRAL-ON

I.   More than 6 months duration
II.   Psychiatric symptoms   - Tearfulness and depression > 4 months
                                   - Suicidal ideation
                                   - Rape-related phobias e.g. agoraphobia
                                   - Interfering with normal life or lasting > 4 months
III. Prolonged sexual difficulty or diminished sexual enjoyment
IV.   Maladaptive response   - drug
                                   - alcohol abuse
V.   "Blocked therapy"
      The "helpless" therapist
      The "burnt-out" therapist
      The victim who demands more time/energy than the GP can provide

Rape victims occasionally present months to years after the
rape, many of them, never having talked about it before. This is
likely to occur when an event in their lives occurs, that serves to
recreate memories of the rape that until then had been thought to
be successfully suppressed. Certain life-events are more likely than
others to cause this reaction:

    Court appearance
    First sexual experience following the rape
    Marriage
    Birth of a child
    Emerging sexuality in female children
    Anniversary reactions[18]

Generally these events can be managed by being sensitive to the special significance of each, in the light of the woman's past victimisation.

It takes time and a certain hardiness to counsel rape victims and is work which, if undertaken seriously, can leave the counsellor feeling vulnerable, helpless and often frustrated. There is little evidence to support the common assertion that rape victims should be counselled by women[19]. It is the attitude of the counsellor towards the victim rather than the gender that is important. Indeed, the early introduction of a sympathetic, warm and trustworthy male figure after a rape can be beneficial.

Even if willing to do this work, the constraints on most GP's time may mean that early referral on is the most appropriate course of action either to psychiatrists or alternative counselling services such as Rape Crisis Centres. There are disadvantages with all these possibilities: the waiting lists for psychiatric evaluation are generally so long that by the time an appointment has been received, the need has passed. In addition, there are very few psychiatrists who are trained, or take an interest in this kind of crisis reaction or the specific problems of rape. Although there is great variability, Rape Crisis Centres generally adopt a feminist approach to counselling rape victims and see rape as an extremist rather than an eccentric act, i.e. an act committed by any man on any woman.

Victim support schemes were set up in the 1970s to help victims of crime and are now found throughout England, Wales and Northern Ireland. They are staffed by trained volunteers who provide both counselling and practical support for rape victims, such as accompanying the victim to special clinics, to the police station throughout the court process. Unlike many Rape Crisis Centres they have both male and female counsellors and will also treat male victims. Although there is no real limit to the amount of time the counsellor remains involved with the victim, the voluntary nature of the organisation means that only a proportion of all referrals can be taken on. The majority of VSS referrals are still via the police, although certain branches are beginning to accept direct referral, particularly if medical back-up is guaranteed.

REFERENCES

1. Dukes R L and Mattley C L (1977). Prediciting rape victim reportage. Sociol. Soc. Res., 62, No. 1
2. Mezey G (1986). Help for the victim of violence. Bull. Br. J. Psych. (in press)
3. Saragin E (1976). Prison homosexuality and its effects on prison sexual behaviour. Psychiatry, 39, 245-257
4. Groth N and Burgess A (1977). Rape: a sexual deviation. Am. J. Orthopsychiatry, 47, 400-406
5. Gebhard P H (1965). Sex Offenders: an Analysis of Types. (New York: Harper and Row)
6. Brown Miller S (1975). Against our Will: Men, Women and Rape. (New York: Simon and Schuster)
7. Burgess A and Holmstrom L (1974). The rape trauma syndrome. Am. J. Psych., 131, 981-988
8. Rado S (1948). Pathodynamics and treatment of traumatic war neurosis (traumatophobia). Psychosom. Med., 4, 362-368

9. Ochberg F (1977). The victim of terrorism: psychiatric considerations. <u>Terrorism: An International Journal</u>, **1**, 1-22
10. Lindemann E (1944). Symptomatology and management of acute grief. <u>Am. J. Psych.</u>, **101**, 141-148
11. Conklin J E (1972). <u>Robbery and the Criminal Justice System</u>. (Philadelphia: Lippincott)
12. Sutherland S and Scherl S (1970). Patterns of response among victims of rape. <u>Am. J. Orthopsychiatry</u>, **80**, 503-511
13. Burgess A and Holmstrom L (1974). <u>Rape: Victims of Crisis</u>. (Bowe, MD: Brady Co.)
14. Symonds M (1976). The rape victim: psychological patterns of response. <u>Am. J. Psychoanal.</u>, **36**, 27-34
15. Shapland J, Willmore J and Duff P (1985). <u>Victims in the Criminal Justice System</u>. (London: Gower)
16. Silverman D C (1978). Sharing the crisis of rape. Counselling the mates and families of victims. <u>Am. J. Orthopsychiatry</u>, **48**(1), 166-173
17. Notman M and Nadelson C (1976). The rape victim: psychodynamic considerations. <u>Am. J. Psych.</u>, **133**, 408-412
18. Renvoize E B and Jain J (1986). Anniversary reactions. <u>Br. J. Psych.</u>, **148**, 322-324
19. Bassul E and Apsler R (1983). Are there sex biases in rape counselling? <u>Am. J. Psych.</u>, **140**, 305-308

95

10

Psychiatric emergencies in children and adolescents

Dora Black

QUICK REFERENCE GUIDE

THE SORTING PROCESS

Most psychiatric disorders in children and adolescents develop slowly and rarely present as emergencies. This chapter outlines the exceptions, and certain situations in which prompt action may avert psychiatric symptoms in children caught up in events they cannot influence or control.

Emergencies may occur in the following:

Emotional Disorders
  Hysteria,
  Acute phobic reactions,
  School refusal,
  Sleep and habit disorders,
  Attempted suicide,
Certain Conduct Disorders,
Acute Psychoses,
Anorexia Nervosa,
Child Abuse,
Sexual Problems.

Situations where preventive intervention may be effective:

Post-Traumatic Stress Disorder,
Life-Threatening Illness,
Bereavement, see Chapter 12B.

HYSTERIA

This can be the most dramatic child psychiatric emergency, and whilst rare, is a common reason for parental panic. A child, or more commonly, an adolescent, reports sudden onset of amblyopia, or goes suddenly off her feet with paralysis of one or both legs. Rarer presentations include severe and intractable pain (especially facial) and pseudo-seizures - the latter is associated especially with intra-familial sexual abuse.

About 50% of children diagnosed as hysteria later are found to have organic disorders - especially in amblyopia. Children with the psychological disorder tend to have a rapid onset, a family history of hysteria, and/or close relative with disease at the same site, "La belle indifference" is uncommon in children.

Recovery from the disability may take time and dramatic cases are rare. Specialist opinion is usually needed and the child is best admitted under a paediatrician to a hospital with good child psychiatric facilities where an early joint approach to treatment can be implemented. Delay in admission usually leads to prolongation of disability as the longer the child is sick the harder it is for him/her to give up the sick-role.

Psychological symptoms such as amnesia, wandering, multiple personality are rare in childhood. However, **epidemic hysteria** is commoner in children in institutions such as boarding schools or hospitals. Symptoms such as fainting, dizziness, pseudo-seizures, shivering, etc. start in one or two disturbed and dominant girls and spread rapidly. It is essential to isolate the key figures rapidly and initiate investigations into the factors in the institution which may be maintaining vulnerability (see also Chapter 7).

ACUTE PHOBIC REACTIONS

Young children take their cue in strange situations from those around them. Most phobic disorders in young children are therefore learned from others, most specifically their mothers. Young children most commonly have phobias about **animals and insects, the dark, thunderstorms** and **death**. Children who have hospital treatment may develop **needle phobia** or phobias to **white coats** (doctors) or a fear of **operations**, etc. Agoraphobia and claustrophobia are rare in childhood but become commoner in adolescents (and see **School refusal** below).

Children may become fearful of sitting on the toilet or of letting go of bodily excretions. Phobic reactions often develop because of coercive, punitive or painful experiences and careful assessment is needed before treatment is instituted. It is rarely enough to treat the child - the mother may need to be freed too from her fears or punitive practices.

Behavioural techniques such as graduated desensitization in vitro and vivo and flooding are effective, within a therapeutic relationship. The practitioner may be able to use his relationship with the family to effect a rapid recovery using such techniques but should refer to a clinical psychologist in a child psychiatry department if unsuccessful. Occasionally the use of medication such as beta-blockers (in the absence of asthma) or rarely clomipramine may be helpful in encouraging a child to take the first steps in facing the feared object, but drugs should not be used except in the context of a behavioural programme and then for the shortest possible period of time.

Phobic disorders in young children usually respond quickly to treatment and may remit spontaneously with time.

School refusal is the commonest phobic condition in school-aged children. The child stays at home with the parent's knowledge but not consent. The condition must be distinguished from truancy (the child is away from school and home, without parent's knowledge or permission) and parental withholding (child kept at home to help with chores, younger children, usually against child's wishes). It may develop insidiously with somatic complaints (the "masquerade" syndrome) which disappear at weekends and school holidays, or present suddenly with panic attacks and overt resistance to going to school. It is commoner in the youngest child and peaks at times of change of school (i.e. school entrance or entry to juniors, or secondary school or move to a new school). There is inevitably family pathology (e.g. maternal agoraphobia) and the child may be reacting to covert threat of or actual loss of parents. It often follows a bereavement or a life-threatening illness in the child. In adolescents it may herald the onset of a more serious condition such as depression or schizophrenia. It is rarely due to specific school factors but these need to be considered.

Most children are helped by a rapid return to school accompanied by both parents if necessary and family therapy to address the family psychopathology. Drugs such as beta-blockers or clomi-pramine have a role in some cases to aid return but should not be used for more than a few weeks unless there is also a depressive underlay. Unless rapid resolution of symptoms is achieved referral to a child psychiatric department is advised. It is important to ensure that the refusal is treated with urgency; as otherwise the cases become chronic and difficult to treat.

A proportion of these children go on to become agoraphobic in adult life.

SLEEP AND HABIT DISORDERS

Occasionally **insomnia** in young children presents as an "emergency" usually because the parent is lacking sleep rather than the child! About 20% of babies do not acquire a nocturnal sleep habit for about 2 years or need very little sleep. They can be taught to stay alone in their cots without waking their parents. This involves shaping behaviour by gradually extending the time they are left alone before the parent responds to their calls. A helpful book for both parents and practitioners is My Child Can't Sleep by J Douglas and N Richman (Penguin 1984) which outlines the techniques to use to help a family with a sleepless child. In an emergency (to let everyone have some sleep) Vallergan Forte (trimeprazine-tartrate) syrup 15-90 mg per day is helpful. Young children tolerate large doses remarkably well.

Whilst **insomnia** is unlikely to present as an emergency, severe **constipation with tenesmus** is not an uncommon emergency presentation in young children. The majority of children who deliberately retain faeces and resist the call to stool have been subject to coercive toilet training and the symptom is often a pointer to serious family psychopathology. **A search for organic factors is important**: anal fissure, (which can be a **result** of passing an inspissated motion as well as a **cause** of withholding) dehydration, lack of fibre in the diet and rarely Hirschsprung's disease.

The practitioner, called as an emergency to a young child can do much to alter family attitudes in a bowel-conscious, perfectionistic family by simple measures. However, in older children the pathology is usually more intractable and family and individual psychotherapy with in-patient admission for retraining may be necessary. Relief of pain and constipation require suppositories, faecal softeners and occasionally enemas. The family and child need reassurance that the bowels can function normally and that retention of faeces for long periods (up to 3 months has been recorded) is compatible with good health and the restoration of normal functioning. The physiological process should be explained and the family must learn to withhold criticism and punishment, rewarding with praise, the child's efforts to comply.

ATTEMPTED SUICIDE AND OTHER DELIBERATE SELF-HARM

Whilst suicide is unknown in young children, deliberate self-harm may occur prepubertally. Some cases of "accidental" poisoning in young children have been shown to have been deliberate and although the concept of death is poorly developed before the age of 8, I have known a child as young as 3 years ingest tablets after her father's suicide in order "to go to daddy". It is rare for the prepubertal child to try to harm herself. Many adolescent suicides (commoner in boys) cannot be prevented because the suicidal act is the first and only manifestation of a serious psychiatric disorder such as manic-depressive psychosis or schizophrenia, but you may avert tragedy by taking seriously depressed mood, sudden school failure or suicidal talk especially after an adverse life event (e.g. bereavement, parental separation or illness) or if there is a family history of depression.

A practitioner called to see an adolescent who has tried to harm herself (it is usually a girl) should not be reassured by the apparently trivial nature of the action. Young people need to be listened to seriously and they and their families may need the breathing space that hospital admission can give. It is recommended that after the first aid (e.g. provoking vomiting) all young people under 16 should be admitted to the paediatric ward of the local hospital following overdose (the most common adolescent self-harm), no matter what the medical findings are. About a quarter of these young people will be found to be depressed and the others will be living in disturbed families or other settings, experiencing many problems especially hostility from their families. Overdosing may be the first manifestation of **intra-familial sexual abuse** (see below), or **schizophrenia**. Less commonly more violent methods of self-harm may be employed, especially by boys, such as **hanging, shooting or jumping from heights.**

The practitioner should ensure that child psychiatric advice is obtained as the treatment for the injury may be in the hands of specialists who work less closely with child psychiatrists than do paediatricians and referral may be overlooked. As in older girls, **slashing of the arms** with razor blades may occur in younger adolescents as a tension-relieving phenomenon rather than with suicidal intent. Suicidal behaviour is learned and may be imitated. Epidemics have occured in institutions.

In all cases of self-harm, the degree of **suicidal intent** and **risk of repetition** must be assessed (see also Chapter 6).

Suicidal talk

A practitioner, called by a parent or teacher when a youngster has been talking about killing himself, must examine his mental state after taking a history. Suicidal feelings occur in about 10% of adolescents but few of them act on them. Enquiry should be made about whether they have done anything before (taken overdose, etc.) and whether they have thought about how they would kill themselves. Well-thought-out plans indicate serious intent as do previous, possibly undetected tablet ingestion. A depressed mood together with a feeling of hopelessness about their situation or the future, or a revelation about sexual abuse are indications for urgent action (hospital admission or social services taking into care, pending investigation).

CONDUCT DISORDER

Although conduct disorders in children and adolescents are common, they will only rarely present as emergencies in general practice, most being dealt with by police, education, social work and probation services - with direct referral to child psychiatric services as appropriate.

Aggression. The commonest condition presenting as an emergency is **physical violence** in an adolescent (who may be physically very strong). This rarely occurs de novo and when it does, organic causes such as **hypoglycaemia, brain pathology** (epilepsy, injury, infection, tumour, dementia, etc.) and **illicit drug taking** (see below) must be excluded. **Psychotic disorders** (see below) especially mania and paranoid schizophrenia, may present with sudden aggressiveness.

The majority of aggressive episodes are however related to long standing personality disorders and family disturbance and need a combined treatment approach using family therapy, behaviour modification programmes, social skills training and attention to learning difficulties. The practitioner, after assessing the situation, separating the combatants and making a preliminary diagnosis will need to call on the services most able to offer an eclectic and broad based approach to treatment.

Running away. If the practitioner becomes involved with an adolescent or child who repeatedly absconds from home or school the possibility of **sexual or physical abuse** must be considered and a careful physical examination will be helpful which will also give him an opportunity to talk with the patient alone. Other causes are **mental retardation, marital conflict** and **parental hostility**. An epileptic or hysterical fugue will result in alteration of consciousness and amnesia.

Illicit drug-taking may result in an emergency call and should be borne in mind whenever an adolescent presents with abnormal behaviour, which may include aggressiveness, paranoia, formication, sleepiness, coma, hallucinations (especially visual) and delusions. The commonest drug in adolescents as in adults is of course, **alcohol**, but rarely does it pose diagnostic problems.

Drugs

The commonest drugs used by young people are **solvents** and **cannabis**. They are usually easy to detect (solvents by the smell and circumoral rash and cannabis by reddened eyes as well as alteration of consciousness). Emergency treatment must be family-orientated and reassuring and calming the parents may be as necessary as sorting out the young person's difficulties. Since adolescents are risk-taking creatures, too extreme a parental reaction may provoke a repetition of what was merely a normal adolescent experiment. If there are problems in the young person's life for which they repeatedly seek a solution in drugs or alcohol, referral for individual or family therapy is indicated.

A psychotic-like condition can be provoked by **amphetamine** misuse ("speed"). It responds to the administration of phenothiazines but the patient may require hospitalization. **Lysergic acid ("LSD")** can cause hallucinations and bizarre behaviour.

Some **prescribed drugs** can occasionally cause psychiatric symptoms. **Anticonvulsants** can occasionally cause psychotic states. **Methylphenidate** can cause depression. Parkinsonian symptoms can occur with **phenothiazines**. **Steroids** can cause psychosis.

Stealing

The practitioner is likely to be called by parents if their child or adolescent has stolen from a shop and is apprehended by the police. Sometimes the hope is that a "medical" excuse will be found. Unless there is a genuine medical condition leading to impaired consciousness, the practitioner's contribution is likely to be to help the parents to accept that it may be helpful that the child has been apprehended sooner rather than later and to explore any family and individual factors which may be acting to produce antisocial behaviour.

Fire-setting

Whilst rare in childhood, repeated and persistent fire-setting is a serious and dangerous symptom and referral for specialist help is essential. However, young children are fascinated by fires and can be taught how to make a "safe" fire rather than being denied the pleasure. A safe fire is one lit in the open on a non-flammable base, away from trees, house and furniture, with an adult present and the means to douse it at hand.

ACUTE PSYCHOTIC REACTIONS

Schizophrenia is extremely rare in pre-puberty and its onset is normally insidious so emergency presentation is unlikely. In adolescence it increases in frequency but still represents a small proportion of psychiatric problems (1-5%). The presentation of schizophrenia in adolescents is similar to adult presentation except that paranoid delusions are less common and anxiety is higher. It may be difficult to distinguish from depression and specialist advice should be sought. The differential diagnosis from drug-induced psychosis and rare organic neurological conditions must be made.

Manic-depressive psychosis. Although this is also rare in childhood and early adolescence, its first manifestations may be acute mania. I have been called as an emergency to the house of a 15-year-old boy who was literally pulling the house down around him in this condition.

Tragically, a completed suicide may be the first indication of a severe depression in an adolescent. Suicidal threats must be listened to and if there is doubt about the diagnosis, specialist referral is essential.

Emergency management of acute psychotic behaviour

Use of a Care Order or ascertainment under the 1983 Mental Health Act may be necessary. The shortage of adolescent psychiatric in-patient beds may necessitate admission to a general psychiatric facility.

Chlorpromazine, by injection if necessary, has sedative and anti-psychotic activity. It is inadvisable to use depot preparations in a newly diagnosed schizophrenic patient because of uncontrollable side effects. Medication should only be given if essential to calm a violent or uncontrollable patient as it may obscure diagnosis.

Referral to a child and adolescent psychiatrist with access to in-patient facilities is essential.

ANOREXIA NERVOSA

The peak incidence for the onset of this condition is in adolescence. It can occur prepubertally when the prognosis is poor. Although the diagnosis is not difficult, it may present as an emergency because of acute cachexia and dehydration, the girl having hidden her gradually deteriorating state by the use of loose clothing. The differential diagnosis is from other wasting disorders - all of which are extremely rare in adolescence. Bulimia is less common in young anorexics but must be enquired for. Typically, the disease starts around puberty as a response to mild (or imagined) obesity. Dieting may have been encouraged by parents and practitioners. If weight loss is not carefully monitored, by the general practitioner, anorexia nervosa may result. The patient is convinced she is overweight in spite of gross emaciation and will exercise and diet when it is dangerous to do so. In extreme cases admission to a paediatric ward with good child psychiatric liaison is indicated. Family therapy has been shown to be the treatment of choice in anorexics still living at home.

CHILD ABUSE

Child abuse can be **physical, emotional or sexual**. Children can be abused by acts of commission or omission (neglect). (See <u>Child Abuse</u> by R Kempe and C H Kempe, Fontana, 1978.) Emergency presentations occur in physical and sexual abuse. The possibility of abuse must be kept to the forefront of his mind if a practitioner is not to miss what **may be a fatal condition**. A one-month-old baby died of cerebral haemorrhage from being shaken by a parent. She had been presented on three occasions in her short life to the general practitioner with bruising and lack of movement of a limb. Skeletal survey post-mortem revealed old (!) fractures. A higher level of suspicion in the practitioner might have saved the child's life.

Common presentations of physical abuse are as follows:

1. Bruising or injuries not consistent with explanations proffered or where there has been an unreasonable delay in seeking treatment.
2. Certain injuries - e.g. facial, finger-tip bruise marks, repeated fractures in babies and young children, cigarette burns, subdural haematoma.

If abuse is suspected, **try to admit the child to hospital**. It is better not to discuss the possibility of abuse until the child is safe. Your suspicions must be conveyed to the duty paediatrician preferably by phone rather than by a note which may be read by the parents. Social Services will be involved and it is helpful if the practitioner can attend the initial case conference as contributing your knowledge of the family will enable the most effective help to be mobilized. **The aim must be the protection of the child from further abuse**.

SEXUAL PROBLEMS

Acute homosexual anxiety may present as an emergency. This is becoming more common because children are exposed to the existence of homosexuality through the media. A child of either sex, suddenly believes or fears that he/she is homosexual, and becomes panic-stricken and unamenable to parental reassurances. This can occur prepubertally but is commoner as young adolescents. It is essential to interview the child on his own and gently ascertain the origin of his fears - probing for possible homosexual abuse inside or outside the family. The most usual precipitants however, are teasing at school - especially if the child is gentle and bookish and lacks assertiveness - and exposure to the media. This is an indication for speedy skilled psychotherapeutic help, if possible, as reassurance alone is usually unsuccessful. If such help is unavailable, the practitioner should take the line that homosexuality is an acceptable outlet for sexual feelings and that love and tenderness are what matters. Exploitation of either sex by either sex is what is unacceptable. So that the young person's sexual orientation is of less importance than the quality of relationships with his peers. In other words, "you fear you are homosexual .... you are too young to have developed an adult sexual orientation yet but whatever that will be is OK, providing ...." etc.

Child sexual abuse

The involvement of dependent, developmentally immature young people in sexual activities they do not understand, to which they are unable to give informed consent or that violate the social taboos of family roles is on the increase; or is the awareness of what has probably always been present, but unacknowledged, increasing?

About one in ten adult females report sexual abuse in childhood, much of it by family members (fathers, stepfathers, grandfathers and older brothers) or by adults familiar to them and who are in positions of authority. Female abuse of young males occurs but is probably rarer - at least by family members. **Children rarely report it and when they do they are rarely lying.** They are more likely to present with symptoms - the significance of which may be missed unless the practitioner has a high level of suspicion.

Common presentations are:

1. **Vaginal bleeding, discharge or soreness.**
2. **Repeated urinary infections.**
3. **Pain in or injury of vulva, vagina, urethra or anus.**
4. **Foreign bodies in urethra, bladder, vagina or anal canal.**

In addition, other symptoms can be present which are not specific to the condition and vary with age:

Bruises and injuries to "sexual" parts of body; i.e. breasts, buttocks, etc.
Attempted suicide.
Pseudo-epilepsy.
An excessive precocious preoccupation with sexual matters.
Under-age pregnancy - especially when the father is not identified.
Older girls who become promiscuous or repeatedly run away.

There may also be general symptoms of disturbance in functioning. Seeing the patient alone and asking if she has been touched by anyone in her private parts (with young children, their names for genitalia etc. must be sought) in a way she did not like will often elicit information. **The prime purpose of diagnosis is protection of the child from further abuse.** Punishment of the perpetrator is of less concern to the practitioner and anyway, evidence sufficient to convict is notoriously hard to obtain in most cases. **If CSA is suspected, the practitioner should refrain from examining the child or voicing his suspicions at this stage but swiftly obtain a competent paediatric or paediatric gynaecological opinion.** Where rape or violent sexual abuse has occurred by strangers, a police surgeon examination as soon as possible will ensure that fresh samples of semen, etc. are properly obtained and the matter should be pursued urgently.

For if the diagnosis is missed, the child (and children as young as one year can be seriously abused) may be condemned to live out her childhood with an abusing parent who feels safe in the knowledge that he has not been detected. The results for the girl are dire. **Prostitution, premature pregnancy, school failure, social ostracism, depression, suicide and an inability to protect her own children from abuse, are all commoner in sexually abused children than their non-abused peers.** Probably a single experience can be coped with. It is the repetitive nature of the experience which is thought to be damaging.

Referral should be made to a paediatrician who works closely with his child psychiatrist and social work colleagues for admission as a matter of urgency (see also p.121).

SCHOOLGIRL PREGNANCY

May result from CSA but can be the result of a relationship with a peer. In these cases the girl is usually more mature than her friends. It is **increasing as the age of puberty goes down** and there is greater sexual freedom in society. Again a high index of suspicion is necessary so that early diagnosis is made and the options for the girl can be discussed. **Pregnancy testing should always be performed when CSA is established in a girl past puberty, in attempted suicide and menstrual irregularities** after a girl is privately questioned tactfully about the possibility of pregnancy. Some practitioners hesitate for fear of giving offence. Not to do so renders the girl less likely to be able to take advantage of the options. Those girls and their families who elect to continue with the pregnancy should be referred where possible to an antenatal clinic specializing in adolescent pregnancy. Special attention must be given to the maintenance of the girl's education throughout pregnancy and afterwards.

Local education authorities often have special facilities and they should be contacted early in pregnancy so proper arrangements can be made.

POST-TRAUMATIC STRESS DISORDER

A child may be adversely affected by traumatic events occurring in his/her family or community. Unless the children are separately considered and steps taken to protect them, they may develop signs of stress and long-term damage may ensue.

In any of the conditions described in the earlier chapters concerning adults as parents, vulnerable children may be affected. In dealing with a psychiatric emergency in an adult the following may lead to post-traumatic stress disorder in the children.

1. **Acute Separation.** If the major caretaker of a child is hospitalized, deserts or dies, or if the child is kidnapped by a noncustodial parent or has to be taken into care, so loses his major caretaker suddenly, he may develop **acute separation anxiety**. This is at its height between the ages of six months and four years. It is mitigated by the presence of familiar people and surroundings.

2. **Acute Fear.** If a parent becomes acutely **psychotic** or **violent** or **self-destructive** - or a parent or child suffers from the violence of others, especially if the child is witness to, but helpless to prevent violence to a parent. If a father kills his wife or a child, this is perhaps the most traumatic of all situations for a child witness but **rape** and other **grievous bodily harm to a parent** or **terrorism** or **natural disaster** in a community can be terrifying to a child caught up in the events. The evidence is that children take their cue from parents and other adult caretakers (teachers, etc.). If they are coping, then the trauma for the child is lessened. Age and stage of development are important mediating influences. Other protective factors are sex (girls are less vulnerable) a stable, warm, supportive family and a flexible temperament. If a child feels a sense of personal power and ability to influence the course of his life, he is less likely to break down under stress. In most of the events described above, the child is a passive witness, unable to act.

Symptoms

1. The repeated reoccurence of the trauma - in play and dreams, sounds and images.
2. Psychic numbing or affective constriction - the child will be very subdued or even mute - or inappropriate detachment.
3. Non-specific symptoms - fear, anxiety, startle reactions, etc. Sleep disturbances, learning difficulties and conduct disorders (especially in adolescents). Traumatic amnesia or denial are rare in children.

Treatment

Recent work from the USA and Israel **has demonstrated the effectiveness of a rapid therapeutic interview** (within 48 hours of the trauma) in which the child is helped initially to express the impact of the trauma in play, fantasy and through metaphor. Mastery of the traumatic anxiety is fostered by a thorough exploration of the child's experience, reliving the trauma, promoting emotional release and then helping him to use cognitive coping strategies to improve his sense of mastery. These techniques are specialized and are not yet well developed in this country. Interested practitioners can consult an experienced child psychologist or psychiatrist or read "Witness to violence: the child interview" by R Pynoos and S Eth (1986) Journal of the American Academy of Child Psychiatry, **25**, 3, 306-319. Because of the emergency nature of the events and the needed response, the practitioner may be the most suitable and available professional person to conduct the interview and prevent the personality constriction that may ensue if the events are not properly dealt with by the child.

CHILDREN FACING LIFE-THREATENING ILLNESS AND DYING CHILDREN

The practitioner may be able to help the child and his family to cope with this most unnatural of situations when a child threatens to predecease his parents. Although psychiatrists and psychologists have developed ways of helping, the introduction of "psychogogues" at a later stage in the disease is often not acceptable to parents and it is helpful if the practitioner can offer psychological help as well as medical care. This involves giving the child an opportunity to understand the nature of his illness and the immediate future picture; i.e. is this an illness which will get better, or not? The child needs time and opportunity to ask about death, and should feel that his doctor is not afraid to talk about such a serious subject. Even quite young children can cope, if he feels people are honest, warm and caring. If death is a possibility in the near future, he needs reassurance that **dying does not hurt** and that **he won't be left alone**.

Parents and siblings need much support and honesty at this time too - they will want to review with you whether they did anything to cause the illness and families with genetic diseases may need special counselling help from a clinical geneticist.

Attention must be paid to financial difficulties caused by the illness, problems of baby-sitting and the neglect of siblings. After a death, siblings often feel guilty about the fact that they "inherit" toys, etc. and about their ambivalent feelings towards the dying child. They may become disturbed and need specialist help.

Fortunately, premature child death is rare but the role of the family doctor in supporting such families is often undervalued.

11

Disturbed adolescents

David Will

QUICK REFERENCE GUIDE

PRINCIPLES OF ASSESSMENT

Adolescence is, under normal circumstances a time of upheaval and change. Normal adolescents are often confusing to the adult, since they may show **swings of mood, exquisite sensitivity** and **oppositional behaviour** that would be regarded as abnormal in an adult. They may also be **very uncommunicative**. It is always important to bear in mind that apparently defiant, paranoid and difficult behaviour may merely be a manifestation of normal adolescence.

Maturational tasks must be accomplished by all adolescents. These are first, the **achievement of independence**: the normal adolescent will progressively emancipate him or herself from home and, by the end of adolescence, will be capable of an independent existence. Secondly, the adolescent must **achieve a sexual identity** and become capable of establishing stable sexual relationships. Thirdly, there is the **achievement of a social and work identity**. The adolescent should develop age-appropriate peer relations and, ideally, settle in an occupation commensurate with his or her ability.

    The assessment of how the adolescent is fairing in the achievement of these maturational tasks is vital. It may provide important clues as to both the nature of the disturbance and to whether the adolescents problems are **long-term or recent**.

The family
Adolescence is often a stressful time for families. Moreover, much adolescent disturbance is either triggered by or is an expression of family disturbance. For this reason it is important to involve parents in assessment.

The community and the school
Adolescents are very sensitive to the influence of their peers. With some types of disturbance, notably delinquency and alcohol and substance abuse, the influence of peers and local community subculture is of great importance.

THE PROCESS OF ASSESSMENT

The adolescent should ideally be seen with both parents. They may first provide vital information about the nature of the adolescent's disturbance, particularly if the adolescent is uncommunicative. Secondly, the doctor may be able to assess family problems that are contributing to the disturbance. The family practitioner is very well placed to do this, since he or she will often have ready extensive knowledge of the family.

What is the nature of the adolescent's disturbance?

1. Is it a **disturbance of conduct** rather than a neurotic or other problem? Are the symptoms violent behaviour, delinquency, running away or oppositional behaviour?
2. Is it a **neurotic disturbance**? Are the symptoms of anxiety or panic, depression or withdrawn behaviour, parasuicide or anorexia nervosa?
3. Is it a **psychotic disturbance**? Are the symptoms suggestive of the adolescent's being out of touch with reality, hallucinating

and behaving in a bizarre way?

4. Is the disturbance indicative of **sexual problems**? If a boy, is he **sexually deviant** and exhibiting himself or cross-dressing? If a girl, is the disturbance suggestive of **sexual abuse**?

How is the adolescent faring in his or her maturational tasks?

If the adolescent is faring well in general, the disturbance is more likely to be an acute response to some obvious precipitant. If the adolescent is not faring well, the disturbance may be but the tip of an iceberg of chronic individual or family pathology.

How is the family functioning?

Does the family seem to be stable and happy or is it unstable and fraught with tension? The nature of the family can provide important clues to the type, severity and optimal treatment of the adolescent's disturbance. For example, have there been recent changes in the family such as, divorce, separation, departure of a family member or bereavement? Adolescents are often very sensitive to such changes and acute disturbance may follow them. The family may, on the other hand, be one with long-standing difficulties such as chronic marital disharmony, or chronic parental illness. Such difficulties may have had a severe long-term effect on the adolescent.

Are there relevant community factors?

These are particularly important in adolescents who present with conduct disorders, especially delinquency. Are they members of gangs? Or, are they involved in a criminal sub-culture or in a drug-taking peer group? This is important to know diagnostically and prognostically, since it is hard for a doctor to compete with the effects of a powerful peer group.

SPECIFIC TYPES OF DISTURBANCE IN ADOLESCENCE

Conduct disorders

There is a generic term given to disturbance whose primary manifestations are a propensity to behave in an anti-social or anti-parental way. There is often a continuity between childhood conduct disorders and adolescent ones, so that conduct-disordered children often grow into conduct-disordered adults. Such adolescents often come from disorganised families where behavioural controls are poor.

1. **Delinquent behaviour** has a peak between the ages of 15 and 16. It rises steadily from the age of 12 and falls away steadily after

111

16. It is far commoner in boys than in girls. Many of the factors that contribute to it are similar to those that contribute to violent behaviour (see below), although peer and community influences are stronger in delinquency as a whole.

Assessment: when a youngster is brought into a doctor's surgery having committed some anti-social act in which the police have become involved, the first basic question is - is the adolescent a socialised or unsocialised delinquent?

i. **Socialised delinquents**

These are delinquents whose delinquent acts are congruent with peer or community values. They tend to commit delinquent acts with others and have good peer relations. As the name suggest, the determinants of socialised delinquency are largely social: such adolescents are following the normal values of a particular sub-culture. At the most extreme, they may be living in a criminal sub-culture, where not to be a delinquent is to be deviant! They may form part of a sub-culture of particular schools with high incidence of delinquency, or be part of a local anti-authority culture of socially underprivileged youngsters.

Family factors may play some part in the production of socialised delinquency. For example, a family history of paternal criminality is of importance and inconsistent behaviour controls or lack of sanctions in response to delinquent activity also play their part.

ii. **Unsocialised delinquents**

These are delinquents whose delinquent activity is not congruent with the values of a peer group. They are often isolated youngsters with poor peer relations and become involved in delinquent activity in response to neurotic or other difficulties (they are sometimes called neurotic delinquents). The delinquent acts are quite incongruent with the culture of their families and often cause great distress to parents. The unsocialised delinquent may present, along with anxious parents as the result of a one-off act of delinquency which appears quite uncharacteristic. Good history taking will usually find a precipitant, e.g. a recent bereavement, a recent conflict at home or school or a pressing anxiety, e.g. fear of pregnancy.

Other unsocialised delinquents may have a delinquent career that is much more longstanding. This may be a response to chronic family stress, e.g. marital disharmony or chronic illness in a parent. Alternatively, the delinquency may have set off a vicious circle whereby an initially insecure adolescent is progressively rejected by his parents as a result of his delinquency and as a result feels more insecure and hence commits more delinquent acts.

2. **Violent behaviour**. Adolescents may present in a surgery following violent acts that they have committed either at home or the
community. These may range from relatively trivial incidents
such as breaking a window to much more extensive occurrences
such as, "smashing up the home", or major physical violence
against other people.

    Assessment: Is the propensity to violent behaviour longstand-
ing or recent?

A. Is the violent behaviour longstanding?

i. **The family factors**
Violent families breed violent adolescents. Thus, if there has
been a culture of violence within a family, the children in
that family are prone to become violent themselves. Children
who suffer child abuse, for example, are at greater risk of
becoming child-abusing adults. For example, an adolesent
may be violent within his own family, turning on siblings or
parents, or may be violent outside his own family, putting
into practise what he has learned in his family context.
Knowledge of the family is therefore essential for assessing
the significance of an act of violence committed by an adolescent.

ii. **Tension-discharge personality**
Such an adolescent will have a long history of conduct disorder with evidence of deviancy, usually present before reach-
ing school. Part of this conduct disorder will be a difficulty
in tolerating frustration and a propensity towards violence.

B. Is the violent behaviour recent?

Recent or "on-off" episodes of violence can be caused by:

i. **Family factors** are once again of great significance. An
adolescent boy may, for example, react violently in response
to such things as his mother introducing a cohabitee into the
family. Such violence may be directed against the mother or
the cohabitee in a sort of a protest. Similarly an acute act of
violence may be a response to a disciplinary act. An adolescent may become so incensed at constraints being placed
upon him that he reacts violently. This may occur more commonly in some single-parent families, where a mother is attempting to bring up adolescent children on her own.

ii. **Alcohol or drugs**
    a.   An adolescent may, when **drunk**, erupt violently par-
ticularly if there has been some source of frustration at
home. Domestic violence under these circumstances is
likely to betoken underlying family disturbances.
    b.   **Solvent abuse** can lead to violent behaviour, both at
home and in the community. There will usually have

113

been some evidence that solvent has been taken, either from its smell on the breath or from physical stigmata, such as red streaking of the face around the nose. Solvent abuse is usually a peer group phenomenon and does not, by itself, indicate serious psychological disturbance. However, solitary solvent abuse tends to be associated with more severe psychological difficulties and also carries a higher risk of mortality, from such things as exposure to the cold and drowning. Solvent abuse is often difficult to treat - particularly if it is being reinforced by the peer group. It is important to know that Evo-Stick (glue) is the safest of solvents used by abusers (see also p.192).

c. Violent behaviour may also occur with **amphetamine** use, and, very occasionally with hallucinogens, such as LSD. It **rarely** occurs with cannabis (see also p.194).

iii. **Temporal lobe epilepsy** is a rare but important cause of recent-onset episodic violent behaviour in adolescents. Parents or witnesses will describe episodes of bizarre, aggressive and sometimes violent behaviour, during which the adolescent does not look himself, has a glazed expression and appears largely unaware of what he is doing. After the episode, there will usually be a post-ictal state. The adolescent will often be able to describe an aura with olfactory or other hallucinations.

iv. **Psychosis** may rarely present with violent behaviour (see below).

v. **School refusers**, in a state of oppositional panic at the suggestion they return to school, may become violent to property or even to their parents (see below).

3. **Runaways**: Adolescents who run away from home often cause great anxiety to their parents and others.
   Assessment: Is this a one-off event, or is the adolescent a repeated runaway?

   a. **One-off runaways**, like parasuicidal adolescents, are often responding to a particular event or crisis. This may be a row with parents, falling out with a friend, or trouble at school. Good history-taking will often reveal the precipitant and may lead to a resolution of the crisis.

   b. **Repeated runaways** are a serious concern since they are usually responding to some chronic stress within the family. As well as more generic stresses, such as marital disharmony, parental violence, (with concomitant fear of corporal punishment), and parental illness, are those associated with a lack of feeling wanted. Thus, some foster children and

114

some adopted children may repeatedly run away from home to test out whether their (foster) parents really want them and will accept them on return. Similarly, adolescents who do not feel secure about parental controls on their behaviour may run away in the hope that this will make passive or feckless parents impose more controls. This strategy often backfires and both unwanted and insecure adolescents succeed only in worrying and then enraging their parents by repeatedly running away. Another important cause of runaways, particularly in girls, is child sexual abuse (see below).

4. **Oppositional adolescents**

Many parents become taxed by their adolescent's oppositional behaviour, which is part and parcel of normal adolescence.

Assessment: Is the oppositionality normal, or does it represent a negative identity?

a. **Normal oppositionality**

It is important to have a good idea of what constitutes normal oppositionality, and to bear in mind the overall maturational tasks of adolescence. If an adolescent appears to be successfully accomplishing these, it suggests that his or her development is not too far awry. Repeated arguments with parents, reluctance to do what is expected of them regarding domestic chores, disputes over clothes, curfews and how much time they spend at home - all these are part of normal adolescence. Added to this, there may be rapid changes of mood and interests, plus a sensitivity to criticism, that parents find quite bewildering.

There are two common situations in which normal oppositional adolescents are referred to the doctor. First, late-developers, who have had a relatively quiescent adolescence until their mid-teens and then, often as a result of new peer contacts, blossom almost overnight into fully fledged oppositional adolescents. This is often accompanied by overswing and the previously bookish scholar will seek to transform himself into a street-wise youngster. Parents and adolescents will usually respond to reassurance and an explanation of what is happening.

The second group who complain about normal oppositional adolescents are parents ill-equipped for adolescence. Two common examples of this group are, first, parents who did not have an experience of normal adolescent oppositionality themselves. Parents from rigid authoritarian backgrounds who were passive and compliant in their own adolescence, can find the normal oppositionality of their own children very threatening. Secondly, parents who themselves had a problematic adolescence may over-react lest their children are going to have the same sort of adolescence as they themselves had. A common example of this is the father who was a delinquent in his adolescence and becomes very anxious lest normal oppositional behaviour in his adolescent children indicate that they too are going to become delinquents.

b. **Negative identity**

This an extreme form of oppositionality in which the adolescent channels all of his or her maturational drives into becoming exactly the opposite of what his or her parents want him or her to be. Thus, the talented and intelligent son of professional parents not only becomes a delinquent, but resolves to drop out of school and work as a labourer. Negative identity represents a maturational cul-de-sac. Very often a negative identity is a response to extreme and/or unrealistic parental pressure over academic achievement. Other factors include overly rigid attempts to make the adolescent mix with the "right sort of friends", or become involved in the "right sort of activities". A negative identity may become extremely entrenched and become very fixed, dominating a youngster's life for several years.

ANXIETY AND PANIC

As a general rule neuroses such as phobias, anxiety neurosis and hysterical neurosis take the same form in adolescents as they do in adults. However, in younger adolescents symptoms tend to fluctuate more than they do in adults and neurotic disorders are less fixed. So, for example, obsessional neurosis is often less enduring in a young adolescent than it is in adults. With increasing age, neurosis in an adolescent comes more and more to resemble that in an adult (see also Chapter 8).

The rest of this section will consider the archetypical adolescent neurosis.

School refusal, a very common cause of anxiety and panic in adolescents. School refusal occurs when a child refuses to go to school, but insists on staying at home instead. (Truants usually pretend to go to school and spend their time out of the home.) In support of this refusal to go to school, the youngster may complain about school - about being bullied, about being picked on by teachers, not liking the buildings - and will almost invariably complain of a plethora of somatic symptoms, such as abdominal pains, ear-ache, headaches, sore throats etc. While at home the youngster will often be content and will frequently be a rather dominant personality of above average intelligence with previously good academic performance. Often the youngster will have been over-protected and over-indulged by one or both his parents, who will often be at loggerheads over the significance of the symptoms. School refusal has a peak incidence in adolescents around the age of 12 or so, usually at the time of transition from primary to secondary school.

It may present in a number of ways:

a. Repeated visits to the family practitioner with a plethora of somatic complaints. These are usually mercurial and no physical cause is found for them. Despite this, the adolescent and often one or both his parents, will complain vigorously about them.
b. **An acute panic attack.** This will often follow an abortive attempt to return the youngster to school. It will quickly resolve if the youngster thinks that no further pressure is being put on him or her to return to school.
c. **"Acute depression" with suicidal threats.** This usually occurs when the youngster realises that his parents or other professionals want him to return to school. He or she becomes acutely distressed, tearful and threatens suicide. The manipulative quality of this "acute depression" is apparent when it quickly resolves if the threat of return to school is withdrawn.
d. **"Berserk" adolescent.** In the same circumstances as c., the youngster, instead of becoming "acutely" depressed, may become "beserk", becoming violent to property and occasionally to persons at home.

Diagnosis is from the history and mental state. Early diagnosis is important, since adolescent maturation can be significantly delayed if school refusal is allowed to persist for a number of years. Any adolescent who is repeatedly missing from school because of a series of vague somatic complaints should be assessed for school refusal.

DEPRESSION, WITHDRAWN BEHAVIOUR, ANOREXIA NERVOSA AND PARASUICIDE

While classical depressive illness is rare in adolescence, many adolescents show symptoms of depression and withdrawal and these may accompany other conditions such as anorexia nervosa, or may contribute to parasuicidal behaviour (see also Chapters 5 and 6).

Assessment Is the depression or withdrawal long-standing or recent?

1. **Long-standing depression or withdrawal can be caused by:**

   i. **Family factors.** Adolescents from emotionally deprived families may be chronically depressed and withdrawn. Examples include families where the mother has a long-standing depressive illness, **or step-families** in which the adolescent has been rejected by a step-parent. Adolescents in extremely over-protective families may retreat from social contact and become withdrawn.
   ii. **Sexual abuse.** Sexual abuse within the family, particularly in girls may be a cause of long-standing depression or withdrawal (see below).

117

iii. **Schizoid personality**. This uncommon condition is characterised by a lack of interest in other people and a
preference to a solitary existence with intense involvement in
fantasy life. It is present from the earliest years and is rare
cause of long-standing withdrawal in an adolescent.

2. **Recent depression or withdrawal** can be caused by:

   i. **Acute family problems** - separation, divorce, bereavement
   and unemployment are common causes of an acute depressive
   reaction in an adolescent whose sensitivity to emotional upset
   in the family may make them a sort of emotional barometer
   for the family.
   ii. **Acute depressive reaction**. This may be precipitated by rows
   with friends, boy-friends or girl-friends, rows with parents,
   trouble at school or fear of pregnancy. It may lead at times
   to parasuicidal behaviour (see below).
   iii. **Anorexia nervosa**. This condition, diagnosed by a triad of
   weight loss, morbid fear of becoming fat and delusional body
   image, is often accompanied by a depressive component
   characterised by feelings of helplessness and uselessness.
   The onset of the rigorous dieting which initiates the anorexia
   nervosa is sometimes preceeded by a period of social
   withdrawal. In the later stages of the illness, depressive
   feelings are common and there may also be obsessional features. Other features include self-induced vomiting; purga-
   tion by laxatives; fanatical exercising and extreme devious-
   ness over matters to do with food. Early diagnosis is important and a careful history should be taken from any adolescent girl with amenorrhea and weight loss.
   iv. **Depressive illness** of an adult type is rare in adolescents,
   but its incidence increases with age. Its diagnosis and prognosis are essentially the same as an adults.
   v. **Schizophrenia** in its early stages may lead to depression or
   withdrawal (see below).
   vi. **Encephalitis**. A rare but important cause of unexplained
   withdrawal or unusual behaviour in an adolescent is an encephalitis. Following a viral illness, the youngster may become
   more withdrawn or show odd behaviour. Standard psychiatric
   history taking is usually unrevealing and, in the early
   stages, there may well be no focal neurological signs. Apart
   from the inexplicable nature of the symptoms, important clues
   to the diagnosis are disorientation, speech and language disturbance, clumsiness and sometimes incontinence. Definitive
   diagnosis is by EEG.
   vii. **Suicide and parasuicide**. Suicide is **virtually unknown before
   the age of twelve**. Although girls attempt suicide more often
   than boys, the ratio of completed suicide for **boys to girls is
   over 2 to 1**. The reasons for completed suicides according to
   notes left by the deceased were, in rank order of frequency: (a) recently getting into trouble, (b) rejection by

boy-friend or girl-friend, (c) fear of a peer, (d) parent's behaviour, (e) feeling of depression, (f) a way out. Almost half of adolescents who commit suicide have previously **attempted suicide and of these almost a third have done so within twenty-four hours of their death**. Suicidal threats or behaviour must therefore **always by taken seriously** (see also pp. 54, 100).

Parasuicide. Parasuicide in adolescents shows many of the same features as parasuicide in adults. It is considerably commoner in girls than boys and is frequently a response to an immediate crisis, such as rows with a parent or a friend, or a boy-friend or girl-friend, or trouble at school. It may also be a way in which problems such as being pregnant are coped with. It is also important to bear in mind that it may be an expression of the fact that the youngster is being sexually abused at home. Youngsters who commit parasuicidal acts also tend to have a higher incidence of physical illness than their peers.

Assessment of a parasuicidal adolescent should encompass both an individual assessment of the youngster and an interview with the youngster and his or her parents and other family members. The importance of the parents' response to the episode is of vital importance and a cold, rejecting response may well indicate that the youngster will attempt to repeat his overdose.

PSYCHOTIC DISTURBANCE

Extreme excitement, elation, depression, delusional ideas, lack of contact with reality, bizarre behaviour and hallucinations have essentially the same causes in adolescents as they do in adults. The commonest type of psychosis in adolescents is drug-induced psychosis (see above). **Psychosis in an adolescent is drug-induced until proved otherwise**.

i. **Schizophrenia** is rare in younger adolescents, but its incidence increases during the teenage years, having a peak in the early twenties. Some adolescent schizophrenics have pre-morbid personalities of the shy, withdrawn, introverted type, while others show no distinctive personality characteristics prior to the onset of the illness. Diagnostic, treatment and prognosis are as in the adult variety.

ii. **Manic-depressive psychosis** is very rare until the late teens. When it occurs it is similar to that in adults.

Rarer causes of apparently psychotic behaviour in adolescence include temporal lobe epilepsy and encephalitis (see above).

SEXUAL DEVIATIONS AND SEXUAL PROBLEMS

Exhibitionism and cross-dressing (transvestitism) are quite common problems in adolescent boys. Transsexualism is very rare and homosexuality is now less frequently seen, as being a problem in its own right.

Assessment: Is the intellectual level of the boy abnormal or normal?

1. **Abnormal intellectual level.** The sexual behaviour of mentally handicapped boys is sometimes socially inappropriate. For example, a mentally handicapped boy may masturbate in public, or make inappropriate direct sexual advances to a girl. This occurs because the boy's socio-psychological development lags behind his physical development. Such sexual misdemeanours do not usually betoken any more profound disturbance.

2. **Normal intellectual level.**

   i. **Exhibitionism.** This consists of exposing the penis, either flaccid or erect, to a member of the opposite sex with a view to shocking or frightening the victim. It is a relatively common condition amongst adolescent boys, but 90% of boys who are convicted for this offence never do it again. The boys are usually somewhat immature, awkward in their social relations with girls and often come from families in which they find it difficult to assert themselves with one or both parents. Their parents are usually highly anxious about the exhibitionism and require reassurance that it does not imply profound sexual pathology in their son.

   ii. **Transvestism** (cross-dressing). This consists of boys dressing up in women's clothing to obtain sexual gratification. It is often a transitional experimental phase in adolescent sexual development and the boys show characteristics somewhat similar to exhibitionists.

   iii. **Transsexualism.** In this very rare condition, the individual feels strongly ("knows" would be a better word) that he or she is the wrong sex. Thus, a boy will feel that he is really a woman trapped, by mistake in a man's body and girls feel the opposite. Transsexuals have a powerful desire to become the opposite sex and many wish to live as the opposite sex, often with the help of a sex-change operation. Transsexualism must be distinguished from simply transvestitism where the individual cross-dresses but has no belief that he is the wrong sex nor a desire to become the opposite sex. Transsexualism has its roots in early childhood and is not amenable to change.

SEXUAL ABUSE OF ADOLESCENTS

Sexual abuse within the family is now being increasingly recognised as a horrifyingly common occurrence. It occurs to both girls and boys, although more commonly to girls. It usually begins when the victim is pre-pubertal, around the age of 8 or 9, and may continue for years. Younger siblings in the family may become involved as well as they grow older. Adolescence is a common age for the victim to complain about being sexually abused. In the first place, the victims now realise the true nature of what has been happening to them and, secondly, the perpetrator's jealousy may lead to the victim being refused permission to go out and mix with boys or girls and this runs counter to the youngster's maturational needs.

Assessment: Is the complaint of sexual abuse overt or covert?

i. **Overt**. Sometimes the victim of sexual abuse will tell someone - a relative, a friend, a teacher, a social worker or a doctor - that she is being sexually abused. The cardinal principle here is that adolescents who say they are being sexually abused are almost certainly telling the truth. Contrary to popular belief "hysterical" accusations are very rare. Consequently, the revelation must be taken with the utmost seriousness and the appropriate action taken.
ii. **Covert**. Much sexual abuse is detected by careful and sensitive interview with a victim who is showing covert symptoms of sexual abuse and who may also be living in a high-risk family. Covert symptoms include many common adolescent problems: suicidal attempts, running away, pregnancy, venereal disease, depression, withdrawal, anorexia nervosa and failing school performance. Any girl showing these symptoms should be asked about the possibility that she is being sexually abused.

High-risk families. The following families are known to have a high incidence of inter-familial sexual abuse: families in which the daughter has assumed the mother's role, families with an ill mother, step-families or other reconstituted families (e.g. with a co-habitee), and families in which one or both parents were sexually abused themselves in their childhood. It is important to stress that such families are not confined to the lower social classes.
Diagnosis is by history-taking, the direction of which will be determined by the index of suspicion derived from the adolescent's symptoms and family background (see also p.105).

12A

The bereaved adult

Colin Murray Parkes

QUICK REFERENCE GUIDE

There is now much evidence[1] that bereavement can have **detrimental effects on both physical and mental health**. On the other hand it can also be an opportunity for personal growth and maturation. The value of the right help given at the right time to those who are at risk has been established in several well-conducted studies of bereavement counselling[2] and the members of the Primary Care Team are often in a position to provide this help.

ANTICIPATION

Bereavements often cast their shadow before and any **help given to the families of terminally ill patients** will do much to mitigate the impact of death. Conversely severe and protracted grief has been shown to follow sudden and untimely bereavements for which people are unprepared[3].

Awareness that a loved person is about to die evokes intense anxiety and a tendency to stay close to the patient. Although this has been termed **"anticipatory grief"** it differs from the grief which follows bereavement in its end result. After bereavement grief eventually leads to detachment from the lost person, in advance of bereavement it leads to increased attachment.

Faced with a coming bereavement **family members need information and emotional support**. Although the information needs to be as accurate as we can make it, we should resist the temptation to predict the length of survival. How often have we heard the expression "The doctor gave him six months to live but...."? Predictions of survival may obsess and haunt the family and since most of them are wrong[4] we would do better to admit our ignorance and help the family to live with the uncertainty that results.

Living with uncertainty places a considerable strain on patients and their families. Regular visits from a trusted member of the Primary Care Team (PCT) can do much to reassure them and prevent the build-up of reflected fear. **Reflected fear** is the fear which a patient sees in the eyes of the people around him. It easily increases the patient's own fear and produces a vicious cycle of increasing tension. Doctors and nurses sometimes add to this fear by signalling their own anxiety or simply by staying away or refraining to talk about the frightening issues that are on everybody's mind.

It takes time to **break bad news** and both patient and family members will want to talk through the implications of any information they receive. The members of the PCT need to support each other in delivering this information in as gentle a way as possible and staying close while it sinks in. Psychological defences protect people from being overloaded with information with which they cannot cope and we should not be surprised if some of what we say is disbelieved, misunderstood or forgotten. It follows that we need to go over the same ground several times and to monitor the other person's perception of the situation.

Some of the **fears of dying patients and their families** are unjustified. For instance many people are more frightened of dying than of being dead. Their picture of "death agonies" may be quite horrific and we should be able to reassure them that we will keep the patient free of pain and give our personal support at all stages of the illness. Likewise, for many people the word "cancer" may mean death in agony and we may have to give very positive reassurance that with current methods of treatment there is no need for pain to remain unrelieved (for a good account of the palliative treatment of late stage cancer see reference 5).

The decision whether or not to encourage a patient to die at home or to enter a hospital or hospice for terminal care, will depend a) upon our ability to relieve physical and emotional distress at home, b) upon the wish and ability of the family to cope, and c) upon the quality of in-patient care available. Home can be the best or the worst place to die.

IMPACT

Although from the patient's point of view, death is often peaceful, for the family it is an awesome and sometimes awful event. Everything that happens, every word or gesture of the attendant doctors or nurses, will become part of a picture that will be remembered for the rest of their lives.

Severe **grief is not an indication for prescribing tranquillisers** or for strict injunctions to "pull yourself together", but a single dose of diazepam will probably do no harm in the event of panic. In most instances the doctor or nurse who stays quietly by until the peak of distress is past and the family are ready to take over, will get people through this crisis in their lives without leaving them with the feeling that they are "weak" or "going crazy".

Family members often need to be reassured that **it is all right to cry** and that there is nothing important that can't wait to be done until they are ready.

Those family members who were not present at the time of death or who wish to do so, should be encouraged to "say goodbye" to the dead person and there should be no rush to get the body out of the home.

Doctors are often asked to recommend the name of a good **funeral director** and it is worth choosing someone who can be relied on to understand the family's needs for support and understanding. Facilities for viewing should be available for any family members who were not present at the time of death and this means that refrigeration should be available.

Whenever **a case must be reported to the Coroner** we need to explain carefully to the family the reasons for this. Families often imagine that there is a suspicion of foul play even when no such suspicion has arisen and the arrival of a policeman to take a statement can be alarming. Most will understand the need for a post-mortem examination in such cases but it is important for the GP to meet with the principal family member whenever a post-mortem has been carried out, to answer any questions they may have and to explain the cause of death. This usually enables us to reassure them that "there was nothing more that could (or should) have been done".

NORMAL GRIEF

Grief is a process, not a state, that is to say there are a sequence of emotional changes through which the bereaved must pass on their way to the new identity that awaits them. Different people will go through the process in different ways and there is **no stereotyped sequence** but the same basic components are present in all cases.

1. The urge to search

In most social animals separation from those to whom they are attached evokes a tendency to cry aloud and to search. The search takes priority over all other activities.

Human beings may be aware that searching for a dead person is pointless, but this does not prevent a strong impulse to do just that. **The pang of grief** is an intense feeling of pining which is accompanied by all the physiological features of intense anxiety and is triggered by any reminder of the loss.

Sufferers exhibit a strong tendency to return to places and objects associated with the lost person and to go over in the mind the events leading up to the death as if, even now, they can find out what has gone wrong and put it right. A clear visual memory and a sense of the presence of the dead person is often cultivated and vivid dreams of their return reflect the search. So too does the tendency to misperceive sights and sounds as if the dead person had come back, "I keep hearing his footfall on the stair and twice I thought he was coming through the front door", said one widow. **Hypnagogic hallucinations,** in which the dead person is seen briefly while the mourner is in a drowsy state of mind, are quite common and the bereaved may need reassurance that these are not a sign of mental illness. These hallucinations disappear as the person wakes up and they are usually dismissed as "my imagination", but some take them as evidence of spiritual contact with the dead and a few are alarmed by them. They are to be distinguished from **horrific memories** of the death itself which sometimes haunt people who have witnessed a particularly harrowing type of death and which contribute to the development of post-traumatic neuroses (q.v.).

2. The urge to avoid searching

Almost the first thing that a mother says to her child is "Don"t cry" and most societies attach importance to the control of all strong emotions. **Western civilisations** have taken this "stiff upper lip" so far that it is no longer possible for people to cry at a funeral without feeling that they are "letting the side down". This inversion of the norm of most societies is a relatively recent development and one which threatens to turn mourning rituals from being a support to the bereaved to an ordeal[6]. Some clergy confound the problem by making it an act of faith for Christians to face bereavement with fortitude. Yet this is surely a time when pining is a natural reaction which needs to be expressed.

The extent to which people feel free to express their longing for the dead person varies greatly. Some cry in public and in private, some cry in private and some not at all. Some treasure reminders of the dead person and fill the home with photographs, others put away all reminders and try to avoid them, a few get rid of everything and move away in the hope of escaping from anything that might evoke a pang of grief.

One way to avoid pining is to **keep busy** and some people fill their time with activities in a conscious attempt to distract themselves. Most however, will reach a compromise. They allow certain times to be devoted to grieving, they visit the grave, talk to their family about what has happened and shed a tear. Then they begin to feel a bit better and shrug off their grief in order to get on with the day-to-day tasks and responsibilities which remain to them.

3. The urge to discover a new identity

Identity is the lasting image which each of us has of ourselves and our place in the world. It includes everything that I take for granted, everything I assume to be true about myself.

This self-image arises out of and is reinforced by my interaction with the world around me. From the day of my birth I have been building up inside my mind an **internal model of the world** around me. Each sensation from the world which I meet (my "life space") is being matched up with this internal world. This enables me to recognise familiar objects - tables, chairs, windows, doors, etc., and to plan my behaviour accordingly. I know where I stand and where I sit.

But my internal world contains very much more than tables and chairs - it contains everything which I assume to be true on the basis of my experience. My wife, my car, my country and my left leg are all part of my internal model of the world. If, as a result of some loss event, I lose one of these things then, for a while, **my internal world will be out of conjunction with my life space**. The amputee who leaps out of bed in the morning to find himself sprawling on the floor, the blind person who strains his eyes in the direction of a sound and the widow who lays the table for two and then realizes that there are no longer two people to eat breakfast - each of these people have acted on the basis of a picture of the world which is now obsolete.

Each time this happens, and it happens even more frequently in thought than in actions, the person is brought up short. Maybe he has lost the person whom he would normally turn to at a time of trouble. Losing that person is the biggest trouble that has ever happened. So the bereaved may find themselves again and again turning towards a person who is not there. "It's like falling down a well, you reach out but there's nothing to grip". Feelings of dislocation or bewilderment result; the familiar world seems to have become unfamiliar, nothing makes sense any more.

Because **we rely on our internal models for our confidence** it is no surprise that bereaved people commonly experience severe loss of self-esteem. It takes time to discover what it means to be a widow or a widower and for a while the bereaved are in **a kind of limbo**.

Most societies allow for this by expecting a **period of mourning**. As at times of sickness, the bereaved are permitted to withdraw from their responsibilities and they are treated with gentleness and consideration by those around them. In many cultures it is believed that the spirits of the dead remain earthbound for a period of time and it is only after a second ceremony that they go to their final resting place. During this period the bereaved are expected to grieve and it is only after the second ceremony, which marks the end of mourning, that they are expected to move on to the next phase of their lives[6]. Van Gennep[7] has referred to these rituals as the **"rites of passage"** and he sees them as important turning points in life. Doctors are often the "ritual specialists" who authenticate a transition and guide people through it.

The **psychosocial transition** which results from a major loss requires the bereaved to review their internal model of the world in order to find out what trains of thought must be revised and what areas remain unchanged. For a while nothing can be taken for granted and it may seem as if every train of thought ends in a blind alley. Slowly and painfully a new railway line is laid alongside the old and the bereaved find new meanings and new directions emerging in their lives. But the old line does not cease to exist and in that sense **grief does not end**. At any time an event which brings that fact to mind can switch a person back onto the old tracks and cause them to re-experience their loss afresh.

This observation detracts from the value of any model of "**stages of grief**", for it implies that grief is never over. But there is, despite this, some point in recognizing the tendency for people to move through a succession of phases even if they move back and forth through these places many times.

The immediate reaction of acute distress seldom lasts for more than a few minutes; this is often followed by a phase of **numbness** before the **pangs of grief** begin. Pangs of grief will usually reach a peak within 5-14 days of a major loss and thereafter they decline in frequency and duration leaving longer and longer periods of **apathy and despair**. At this time the bereaved are more able to accept the reality of the loss but they have not yet found **new directions** in their lives. These emerge in the final phase of grieving along with the resurgence of appetites for food, sex and other interests.

The passage through grief is seldom smooth. Periods of stagnation are followed by turning points when things suddenly improve and much depends upon circumstances and supports.

DETERMINANTS OF OUTCOME

Research has revealed many of the factors that can help or hinder the process of grieving and the development of a new identity. Some of these exist before bereavement, some at the time it occurs and others afterwards.

1. Before bereavement

Previous experience of bereavement can prepare someone for later loss or undermine their ability to cope. Anything which has impaired a person's basic trust in themselves or others will make it more difficult for them to cope with later losses. **Previous psychiatric difficulties,** alcoholism or suicidal attempts should be taken as signs of vulnerability.

The **relationship with the dead person** is all important. Problems are most likely to arise if the bereaved has been excessively **dependent** on the partner or if the relationship has been marred by quarrels and **ambivalence**.

Cultural patterns and religious beliefs which add meaning to death and provide social sanction for grief can be helpful; they may also ensure that members of particular groups are supported in their grief by clergy and others of their faith.

2. Mode of death

Sudden and untimely deaths give rise to reactions of disbelief and a syndrome of lasting anxiety, despite fantasies of continued relationship with the dead. **Protracted death in which the bereaved have played a major part in caring** for a sick person may leave the survivor without roles and with a sense of guilt at having failed to keep the person alive.

3. After bereavement

The **absence of a family which is perceived as helpful** and supportive or of any useful or significant role in life, will reduce the chances of recovery. Pressures from family or work which leave the bereaved with **no time to mourn** may also interfere with the course of grieving.

MALADJUSTMENTS

These factors may act to prevent people from grieving or to prevent them from stopping grieving. Hence **grief may be delayed, avoided or chronic**. At times there may be an increased **risk of suicide** and caregivers should never hesitate to ask, "Has it been so bad that you have wanted to kill yourself" if they suspect that this may be so. Such questions will never precipitate suicide (the bereaved are bound to have thought of it already) but it may enable a life to be saved.

COUNSELLING IN EARLY BEREAVEMENT

While it is important not to make people more worried about their health than they already are, **a visit from a member of the PCT one or two weeks after bereavement** is often helpful and will always be welcomed by the bereaved. Far from intruding on private grief we shall usually find that **people are longing to unburden themselves**. After all there may be nobody in the family to whom it is safe to talk. "We're all bereaved you see", said one widow whose whole family were trying hard not to upset each other.

It is important to **encourage people to grieve** both by asking them about their feelings and reassuring them, when they begin to cry, that this will probably do them good. **Angry feelings** are better expressed than stifled and we should not be in too much of a hurry to defend ourselves or others when anger seems illogical. **Guilt** too may need to be expressed and, if unjustified, its probable origins explored; if justified the person may need to be challenged to find some better way of responding than by castigating him or herself.

Both anger and guilt can have good as well as bad consequences and the aim of counselling should not be to discount them but to help the other person to find a creative use for all this distress.

Grief and its somatic accompaniments may give rise to **fear for one's physical and mental health** and these fears may then aggravate the problem. A clear explanation of these effects with very positive reassurance that "You are not dying of the same disease that your spouse had", or "heading for a nervous breakdown" will break this vicious circle and may lead to dramatic improvement.

Bereaved people may need to be warned not to abuse alcohol or any other drugs which they may be taking for their nerves. On the whole it is better to avoid prescribing psychotropic drugs and in particular the benzodiazepines which easily give rise to habituation in this situation. The bereaved widow or widower is likely to have to sleep in an empty bed for the rest of their lives and the sooner they get used to it the better. Likewise the use of cigarettes for tension reduction will only aggravate any health problems that may arise and people may need to be warned to keep their consumption down.

IN LATER BEREAVEMENT

We need to be on the look-out for people who are "stuck" in their grieving or who are developing fresh problems. **Avoided or repressed grief** may present in the form of hypochondriacal or psychosomatic symptoms, unexplained depression, nightmares, sleeplessness by night, persistent tiredness by day or generalized anxiety. A careful history will usually elicit the fact that the person has never accepted the reality of the loss or experienced grief. Often life will have become filled with frenetic activity to the point of "burn-out" at which point **depression may follow**.

Treatment consists of several interviews at which the person is encouraged to talk in detail about the lost person and the events leading up to his death. **"Linking objects"**, e.g. photographs and mementoes, can be discussed, and anything that has been "put away" brought out. If people have not yet visited the grave they should be encouraged to do so and the therapist may choose to accompany them or advise them to take a tape recorder on which they can record their thoughts and feelings for discussion at the next meeting.

This form of **"guided grief"** can be expected to reduce avoidance and help people through to a better adjustment[8].

Chronic grief is more difficult to treat. Such patients have usually been very **dependent** on the dead person and although they will talk endlessly about their bereavement and always seem better at the end of a session, the improvement does not last. After a while the therapist may begin to feel that the patient has become dependent on him! "You're the only one who understands me, doctor."

This sorry situation can be avoided if we acknowledge at the outset that **the aim of treatment is to help the patient to find new directions** and interests and to say "Goodbye" to the dead person.

At the end of each session, targets to be accomplished by the time of the next visit need to be agreed with the person and written down on the understanding that "I can only help you if you will help yourself". Nothing succeeds like success and the therapist should be as delighted as the patient when new things are accomplished. (After all we are probably the only people in the world who know how much courage it has taken this patient to go through the check-out counter at the supermarket or invite her sister to dinner etc.) Reasons for failure need to be carefully examined before we decide whether to discontinue treatment. Perhaps we expected too much or some unexpected happening may cause us to set a lesser task for next time. But it must be clear to the person that we do take these tasks very seriously.

The final test comes at the end of therapy when it is the **separation from the therapist** that must be anticipated. Grief is an understandable reaction and it is best to set a date for ending well in advance so that there is time for this to take place.

For many bereaved people loneliness and the need to find their way into the world of the bereaved can best be alleviated by **introducing them to an organisation** which can help them. Local circumstances vary but consideration should be given to **Cruse,** which is no longer confined to widows, to the **Compassionate Friends** (for parents who have lost a child), and to **Age Concern** (for the elderly).

REFERENCES

1. Osterweis M, Solomon F and Green M (1984). <u>Bereavement: Reactions, Consequences and Care</u>. (Washington, DC: National Academy Press)
2. Parkes C M (1972, 2nd Edn. 1986). <u>Bereavement: Studies of Grief in Adult LIfe</u>. (London: Tavistock & Harmondsworth: Pelican)
3. Parkes C M and Weiss R S (1983). <u>Recovery from Bereavement</u>. (NY: Basic Books & London: Harper and Row)
4. Parkes C M (1972). Accuracy of predictions of survival in later stages of cancer. <u>Br. Med. J.</u>, **2**, 29-31
5. Baines M (1981). Care of the dying: drug control of common symptoms. <u>World Medicine</u>, November 14th
6. Rosenblatt P C, Walsh R P and Jackson D A (1976). <u>Grief and Mourning in Cross-Cultural Perspective</u>. (NY: HRAF Press)
7. van Gennep A (1960). <u>The Rites of Passage</u> (trans. M B Vizedom and G L Caffee) (Chicago: Univ. Chicago Press)
8. Mawson D, Marks I M , Ramm L and Stern R S (1981). Guided mourning for morbid grief: a controlled study. <u>Br.J.Psychiat.</u>, **138**, 185-193

12B

The bereaved child

Dora Black

QUICK REFERENCE GUIDE

INTRODUCTION

The responses of children to the death of someone close depends on their stage of development, their degree of dependency on that person, the suddenness of the death, how they are prepared and told, who cares for them subsequently, the quality of substitute care and subsequent experiences.

Babies and young children are attached to their major caretakers (usually their parents) and the attachment is mutual and is probably biologically determined as it occurs in all mammals. (See J Bowlby (1969) <u>Attachment</u>, Hogarth Press, for a full account). Disruption of attachment bonds by separation (temporary or permanent) has profound short-term effects on infants and toddlers. Whether it has long-term effects depends on the availability of other familiar figures, the suddeness and permanence of the disappearance, and factors such as age, temperament, intelligence, previous adverse experiences and quality of subsequent care. (See M Rutter (1981) <u>Maternal Deprivation Reassessed</u>, 2nd Edn, Penguin.)

When a child loses a parent by death, short-term distress (grief) occurs in the majority although its manifestations differ with age and experience and are mitigated by the presence of the other parent. Adolescents' reactions are similar to those described for adults above. School children may show no overt grief and are more likely to develop somatic complaints, difficulties in school attendance and behavioural problems. Toddlers may have catastrophic reactions with insomnia, nightmares, withdrawal, anorexia, temper tantrums and may run away "to look for Mummy". Regression in speech and continence with clinging and reluctance to separate from familiar figures is common.

At this age, children often assume a responsibility for the death because of egocentrism coupled with the accident of feeling angry with a parent at the time of death. Babies may react to strange caretakers by failure to feed, and irritability but should respond to patience, gentleness and persistence.

The stages of grief as described above can occur in children too, as young as 18 months but children cannot grieve if they do not know that a parent has died, and do not understand what death means. Mentally handicapped children clearly function as their mental age in respect of bereavement. Much of the long-term distress of children (and various studies have shown that approximately half of all bereaved children have significant impairment of development and function 1-3 years later) is related to failure in those around them to help them to understand what has happened and to express their grief, and share in the mourning, as well as failure to ensure adequate care and protect them from subsequent adverse experiences (prolonged depression in surviving parent, assumption of guilt for death of parent, loss of income, status, home, friends, school, etc.).

A practitioner who enjoys the trust of young families in his practice will encourage parents of young children to give them opportunities for enjoyable brief separation (nursery school, visits to grandparents, overnight stays with friends, camping trips with cubs, etc.) so that if disaster strikes, the child's previous experience of coping without parents and relating to other caretakers, will innoculate him and enable him to cope better with the enforced separation.

PREPARATION AND EXPLANATION

The concept of death grows slowly in children and the adult components i.e. irreversibility, universality, qualitative differences from the living (immobility, decomposition, etc.) and causation (natural as opposed to unnatural) are not fully acquired in the child of normal intelligence until about 8 years of age. Young children's cognitive limitations therefore make preparation difficult but more often preparation is avoided, even when it is possible because of a wish to spare a child's distress, or a fear on the part of the adult of not being able to cope with the child's reactions.

In sudden and unexpected death of a parent, early opportunity for discussion and explanation with the family doctor is essential.

Children should be told early if a parent is seriously ill that he/she "may not get better although the doctors are trying hard to help". Depending on the development of the disease, the time scale and the age of the child, he should be led gently to an understanding that "Mummy is so ill that the doctors can't make her better, although they can make sure that her illness is not giving her pain", and eventually that "Mummy's illness is getting worse, its difficult for her to eat, breathe, stay awake, etc. One day she will die. We will all feel very sad because we will miss Mummy very much but Mummy won't feel anything more because dead people can't feel". (or if religious "Mummy's body will be dead but her soul/spirit will be with God who will look after her"). He needs reassurance that dying doesn't hurt.

Young children have difficulty with religious concepts such as "God", "heaven", "spirit". This is because an understanding of abstract ideas does not develop much before puberty. They will tend to concretise these concepts and be bewildered by them. Concepts such as "spirit" may be equated with ghosts and they may develop nightmares or fears of being watched or haunted by invisible figures. If such ideas are to be given to children they are best given by someone who is a believer himself. Many parents whilst being atheists or agnostics themselves attempt to "explain" death using religious concepts which they do not believe.

The child senses the ambivalence and becomes more, rather than less, confused. Even for believers, simple ideas are best. It is sufficient to say that God will look after Mummy, rather that that "God (or Jesus) loved Mummy so much he has taken her to be with him" thus convincing the child that **his** love was insufficient to keep Mummy here, or that he is in competition with a cruel and powerful being who acts seemingly capriciously.

The reasons for burial and cremation are less difficult for children than they are for some adults. Young children can understand, with help, that when anyone dies (human, animal, plant) the body decays because life is no longer in them to renew the substance. They can be helped to understand that when they cut themselves the wound heals because new skin grows but that does not happen when there is no life left. So the body must be returned to the substances of which it is composed by burying or burning. The mother they knew will be in their minds and memories (and her spirit will be with God for the religious). They can be taught that the "real" person requires a body when she is alive but doesn't need it when she is dead, just as they don't need their shoes when they are in bed, or outgrow their clothes and then dispose of them. The body, when dead, cannot feel, any more than shoes or clothes can.

The practitioner is often in a good position to help a child to understand and prepare for the death of a parent, grandparent or sibling. The religious (or non-religious) views of the family should be respected and the family should be encouraged to talk together about the death or impending death, with the practitioner present to support, help and explain where necessary.

SUBSTITUTE CARE

When it is clear that an illness in a caretaker (usually mother) is going to be prolonged or terminal, it is helpful if a practitioner can take time to discuss with the parents and other relatives, as appropriate, how the children will be cared for. Babies and young children need continuity of care, to ensure their security and mental well-being. Older children (over 5) need to be cared for but can adapt to changes of caretaker or breaks in continuity providing they remain in touch with familiar people and are given explanations of what is happening.

When a mother of a young child becomes ill, the child's immediate care is usually met by father or grandparents. In the absence of suitable available relatives, the local authority social services department may be able to supply an emergency caretaker who can live in or at least care for the child in his own house while father or grandmother is at work. The practitioner, with his knowledge of child development and an understanding of attachment is often well placed to help families find the least detrimental solution for the children and help them avoid making decisions which increase the child's distress (multiple caretakers, removal from familiar surroundings or people, unnecessary changes of routine, etc.).

If the mother of a young child enters the terminal phase of her illness, this should be anticipated and a permanent or long-term substitute caretaker arranged so that the young child can be handed over gradually.

This might be an aunt, grandmother, older sister, a nurse in a day nursery, or may need to be a registered child minder or even foster parent. A young child (under 5) needs the security of a firm attachment to a caretaker who looks after him for a substantial part of the day. Make-shift arrangements should be avoided. Even if the father or grandmother cannot permanently take care of the child full time, he/she should arrange to take time off from work to ensure that the handover to the new caretaker is gradual and smooth.

If a mother of a young baby is admitted to hospital suddenly and there is **no-one** to care for a baby (single parent, father absent, etc.) it may be possible to arrange for admission to the paediatric ward of the same hospital until more satisfactory arrangements can be made. Again, the practitioner will be needed to suggest and arrange this and to ensure the baby and mother have as much contact as her illness permits.

A bereaved father or mother may need considerable help in child-care tasks until his/her grief has abated. Evidence is accumulating that a young child reared by a depressed caretaker can be impaired in his development and learning. The widow or widower needs some time and space to grieve, but young children need to spend a substantial amount of their day with non-grieving caretakers.

SHOULD CHILDREN VISIT A DYING PARENT IN HOSPITAL?

Parents (and hospital staff) often discourage the visit of a child to a very sick parent on what seems often to be good grounds. "The parent is too ill to cope with a young boisterous child", or "the parent is so changed by the illness, or so frightening in appearance because of scars, bandages, tubes, machines, etc. that the child will be distressed", or "the ward cannot cope with noisy young children because of other very sick patients", etc.

On the other hand, if a parent dies before a child has seen him/her and experienced the reality of the changed appearance or lack of ability to cope with the boisterousness or noise, then the process of mourning will be impaired and the child may not be able to accept that the parent **has** been ill and is dying or has died. Clearly children must be prepared for what they will experience before they go to the hospital. But to deny them a last chance to see a parent just because she is too ill, may impair severely their chances of adjustment after the death. This is true of children of any age after about 18 months. It may be necessary, to protect other patients, for the meeting to occur in a side room. The practitioner's help in arranging the visits and in accompanying the children to help them to understand and cope with the experiences is invaluable. Although this is time consuming, the comparative rarity of premature parental death means that the task will not be a frequent one. It is doubtful whether anyone else can perform this function as well as the family doctor, familiar to children and parents, and au fait with hospital procedures, illness and death.

SHOULD CHILDREN GO TO THE FUNERAL?

Practitioners are commonly asked this question, and there is no pat answer. The family attitudes must be explored. The crisis of bereavement is not a time to introduce new and difficult ideas to people. Children of any age over 3 or 4 can benefit by attending a funeral although the first funeral they attend should preferably not be that of a parent, so that they can learn the practices and rituals of their community without having suffered a loss themselves. If a young child attends the funeral of an important and much loved member of their family (parent, sibling, etc.) they should only do so after preparation and in the company of a known adult less affected by the death - the parent of a school friend or a teacher perhaps, so that their questions can be answered and they can be taken home if others' emotions overwhelm them.

Older children and adolescents should be allowed to choose whether to attend; can be encouraged if they are uncertain but not forced to go unwillingly. In some religions the eldest son of a dead man has ceremonial duties to perform and may take some pride and comfort from carrying them out.

Adverse reactions to attending funerals have been reported but are unlikely if preparation and a suitable companion are arranged.

THERAPEUTIC INTERVENTION

Because of children's limited understanding and their dependence on their major caretakers, pathological reactions to parental loss are more frequent in children than in adults. Therapeutic intervention before the death and after in which the whole family takes part, with the aim of facilitating the expression of grief, and the understanding of the illness and death as well as helping the parents to make realistic plans which are the least detrimental ones for their children, and to mobilize available services have been shown to lessen subsequent disorder, at least in the short term. It may be sufficient to support and help the parent who will then be able to encourage his children to express and work through their grief. There is a strong association between the state of the surviving parent's mental health and that of his children. Adolescents, especially the eldest child of the same sex as the dead parent, may assume a parental role and need special help in freeing themselves in order to develop autonomy.

Preventive intervention can most appropriately be done by health visitor or attached social worker, psychologist, community psychiatric nurse or counsellor, depending on the resources of the practice. Consultation and in-service training should be available from the child and adolescent psychiatric service.

A child who persistently assumes responsibility for the death or who is depressed, failing at school or otherwise disturbed and who is not recovering should be referred to a child psychiatric service for more specialized help.

OTHER AND SPECIAL BEREAVEMENTS

Loss of sibling poses special problems for a child. Sibling rivalry is over, and the survivor has "won". Parental attention, lost if the sibling had a long illness, is restored. Yet a playmate has disappeared forever and if the number is reduced from two to one, loneliness and a feeling of being an intruder in the adult relationship is often present. Children may feel that their envy of parental attention in some way "caused" the death of a sibling. They may fear retaliation or even that they may develop the same disease. In some families with familial diseases such as the lipodystrophies, etc. this may be true. If the sibling has been a donor (as in bone marrow transplants) he may believe his marrow was deficient or lethal. Such families are more likely to need specialist help.

Other deaths of grandparents, neighbours, friends, teachers, even pets may affect children disproportionately to their apparent involvement. This may be related to fantasies which will need careful exploration. For example, a 4-year-old whose friend's mother died developed acute separation anxiety which was only relieved when her fear of her mother meeting a similar fate was uncovered and dealt with.

Violent death. The death of a parent by suicide, murder or manslaughter poses special problems. If the father kills mother, the children will lose both parents suddenly and in extremely distressing circumstances. They may even be witnesses to the killing. In the case of suicide, they may have been exposed to a mentally ill parent (depressed, schizophrenic) for some time previously. These cases are rare enough and complex enough to deserve the greatest expertise available. A senior and experienced consultant child psychiatrist should be consulted. Social services will usually be involved but both the social worker and the family practitioner are (fortunately) unlikely to have had previous experience of a similar nature. Decisions about the future care of the children should not be made without expert consultation. In the case of murder, rarely are relatives suitable to assume care of the children because of the intense emotions aroused by murder and the hostilities it provokes. The children will need immediate expert help to prevent post-traumatic stress disorder (see Chapter 10) and should be referred as an emergency to a child psychiatric department with a special interest in helping children in crisis.

OTHER LOSSES

Because of their lack of experience, their limited understanding and their great dependency, young children are particularly vulnerable to losses of all kinds, and need to be prepared for them if possible, and supported through them. This includes loss through parental divorce and separation (although they may benefit if parental conflict also lessens - a not invariable concomitant of parental separation!), reversals of family fortune, changes of home and school (although gains may outweigh losses), and loss of limb or bodily function.

CONCLUSION

The death of a parent is probably the most potentially stressful experience of childhood. Fortunately it is rare, and with appropriate support, preparation and therapy, most children will cope. They are most vulnerable at certain ages and when there is sudden and/or violent death. The long-term outcome of bereaved children indicates that most are unscarred by the experience, but the incidence of depression as adults is approximately twice that of non-bereaved and they may, if grief is unresolved, remain vulnerable to loss in future. The death of a parent should be regarded as a child psychiatric emergency and the general practitioner, his team and the child psychiatric service of the community all have a valuable part to play in preventing and mitigating short-term and long-term disorder.

SERVICES AVAILABLE TO THE BEREAVED CHILD AND FAMILY

1. CRUSE - the national organization for the widowed and their children:- counselling and other support services, literature. Branches in most parts of Great Britain. 126 Sheen Road, Richmond, Surrey, 01-940-4818.

2. Child psychiatric departments, child guidance clinics, local authority social services departments, Family Welfare Association. Many have family therapists, individual psychotherapists, counsellors and can offer consultations to families or professionals.

3. Foundation for the Study of Infant Deaths offers counselling services to families including siblings where cot deaths have occurred. 4 Grosvenor Place, London SW1. Tel: 01-235-1721

4. **Self-help groups of parents:**

    a. Leukaemia Society, PO Box 82, Exeter, Devon EX2 5DP. Tel: 0392-218514
    b. Society of Compassionate Friends, 6 Denmark Street, Bristol, BS1 5DQ. Tel: 0272-292778
    c. Other self-help societies where a child has died e.g. Still Birth and Neonatal Deaths Association, Argyle House, 29-31 Euston Road, London NW1. Tel: 01-833-2851
    Multiple Sclerosis Association, 25 Effie Road, London, SW6 1EE. Tel: 01-736-6267 etc. offer help.

5. **In London**

    a. Elizabeth Raven Memorial Fund - Institute of Family Therapy (London), 43 New Cavendish Street, London, W1M 7RG. Tel: 01-935-1651. A charity offering family therapy to families facing life-threatening illness or who are newly bereaved.
    b. Tavistock Clinic, Belsize Lane, London, NW3. Tel: 01-435-7111. An NHS clinic specializing in various forms of psychotherapy.

13

Vulnerable students

John S Munro

QUICK REFERENCE GUIDE

EMERGENCY PRESENTATION

Always look for the circum-oral pallor, frequently present and receding with effective management.

Acute reactive "unhappiness" or "depression"

55% of students refer themselves, usually after discussion with friends. Sometimes the stress of separation from home can only be relieved by brief "repatriation". More often an accumulation of stresses will finally present in a flood of tears - a bed in a quiet corner, tea and a sympathetic nurse together with a mild sedative will give the opportunity to explore and ventilate. The alert physician must be wary of "I took some aspirin for headaches" or "I have buzzing in the ears" - a high index of suspicion for overdoses makes a casualty referral for stomach wash-out imperative.

Work panic and examination stress

33% of consultations are work related, frequently appearing as acute anxiety covering inadequate techniques and responding to appropriate counselling. Immediate examination stress will quickly respond to firm management, separate rooms specially set aside, and the administration of a very short-acting benzodiazepine such as oxazepam 15-30 mg (see also p.74).

Colleague referrals

Anxiety is infectious and calls from anxious colleagues on the staff usually herald an urgent referral - the advantage of hearing an in-depth appraisal from a close but senior contact of the student, gets the physician off to a useful start and may also assist in therapy.

Less frequent presentations are:

Relationship break-up

It is important never to minimise the importance of this event, a common cause of overdoses. They may have to be dealt with in some depth immediately and prescribed for with extreme caution. We, none of us, learn to make relationships easily and no-one teaches us, so learning and its mistakes can be painful.

The morning after

Again, some "accidents" are not included in first-aid manuals but urgent requests for help in the area of contraception have an emotional component as well as a physical need. Besides the appropriate contraceptive medication it is useful to supplement the clinical assessment with some relationship appraisal. Follow-up handouts are useful.

The manipulative episode

Occasionally one's telephone starts ringing and information concerning a distressed student emerges from different sources - each feeling as if being compelled to some kind of action. This "Vesuvius eruption" can be quite dangerous and usually means severe and confused anxiety or an acute behaviour problem. Almost invariably an immediate hospital admission or despatch to home, accompanied, will give the opportunity for a more effective intervention.

The manic episode (see also p.6)

Can and often does occur without any previous morbid history, excluding drug abuse. This can be a frequent presentation of the psychotic disorders in this age group and responds to the administration of chlorpromazine orally or by injection (50-100 mg).

The diabetic

This does rarely present as a paranoid, hostile and confused student, the result of insulin overdose or inadequate diet - intravenous glucose and, if necessary, a few stalwart policemen are effective!

GENERAL REMARKS

Students in common with other young people share many similar problems - in some important respects they differ.

Social

Students tend to be immature - there is little doubt the attainment of good "O" and "A" level grades centres their lives, and leisure and social activities take a more peripheral place.

Emotional

In a similar way the emotional needs are displaced or delayed, or even substituted for in this late adolescent - frequently the identity crisis occurs whilst at University identified by the student as "second year blues", "who am I?", "where am I going?". Yet in a strange way the contrast is heightened as the age of physical maturity becomes younger.

Medical

No one can doubt the effect of education, particularly at parental level, on health care in this very intelligent section of the community - one third of all students wear spectacles, teeth are almost uniformly well cared for - chronic medical problems effectively controlled, e.g. asthma, diabetes, epilepsy, etc. Certain implications of this will be dealt with later.

Academic

One in four young people go on to further education. Students represent the top 3% of the population in intellectual performance. Some achieve this on a high level of anxiety and all are exposed to a prolonged learning stage in their lives.

Dynamics of success and failure

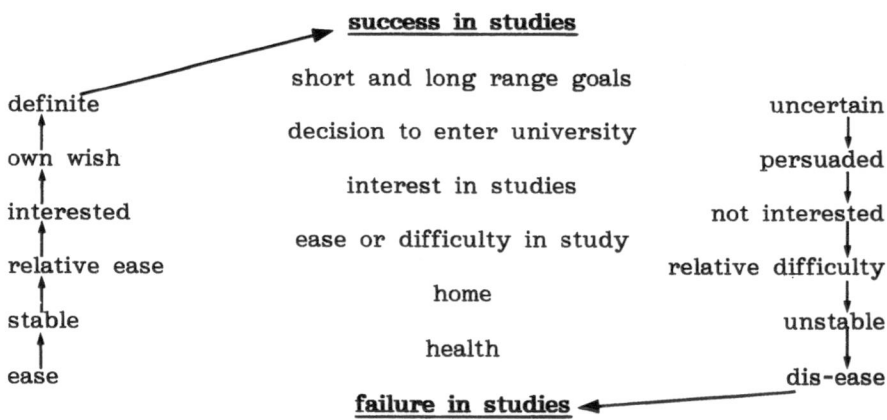

success in studies

	short and long range goals	
definite		uncertain
own wish	decision to enter university	persuaded
interested	interest in studies	not interested
relative ease	ease or difficulty in study	relative difficulty
stable	home	unstable
ease	health	dis-ease

failure in studies

Factors on the right tend to pull towards failure

Borrowed and freely adapted from paper presented by:
Wankowski, J. (1969) Some aspects of motivation in success and failure at university. **Research into Higher Education 1968** Papers presented at the Fourth Annual Conference of the Society for Research into Higher Education. (SRHE)

NEEDS

Needs are important to identify and be aware of.

Curiosity

As one senses that some children are born curious this feature assumes high importance in students - they are trained to ask why and to find out. They make difficult patients demanding time and the reasons, they are articulate and verbal almost into minutiae in terms of symptoms and particularly in their own responses to treatment. Universities tend to over-select the more obsessive introvert students as they tend to achieve higher grades.

Understanding

All young people demand this, yet it is so difficult to offer with any honesty - to understand and be understood is a frequently heard statement, to try should be the response.

Transfer

Perhaps the single most important event for the young person is the move away from home, often for the first time bar holidays, unsupported by parents. The first four weeks of first term at University can be crucial. Drop-outs occur most frequently in this period of time and if efforts by tutors, family doctors and student health physicians can be tuned into this vital period, a great deal can be achieved. The student can be usefully counselled and advised to visit home at frequent intervals so lessening the separational anxiety.

Mature

It is difficult to find a better word to describe the need for a student to accomplish in the short space of 2 years and 9 months at college, a task which other youngsters will have from the age of 16 to complete. Society will expect him to emerge from his degree course a "fully fledged adult". This process can therefore be explosive for some or ducked completely by others with consequences for the caring agencies that operate on campus.

Test out authority

Very many of these young people are going to assume positions of responsibility in later life (most of our Members of Parliament are graduates) - they will need to familiarise themselves with the rules within which Authority functions - many will seek to challenge these for themselves - many revolutions in fact start with campus uprisings!

Degree status

It is not surprising, in the face of these needs, that for a small proportion achieving a degree may seem to be the last thing to do! Yet very frequently the problems present as some difficulty with work and motivation solely or these may front some more serious difficulty.

Grant

It is well to keep in mind that students are a very low income group, indeed two-thirds qualify for exemption from prescription charges. Whilst a few students frequently convey an overall "media view" of this group, it is important to reflect that up to 60% do not receive the full parental contribution and therefore difficulties with lodgings, food and books do arise, aggravated by failure to budget efficiently.

MEDICAL STATUS

In a simple questionnaire administered to all students prior to arrival at University, a distribution of experienced health/disorder is constantly present. About a third return a bland "nil return", about 16% will request further inoculation or vaccination procedures. A history of allergy exists in 11% with penicillin being responsible for more than half. In 9% of students there is a history of personal stress or psychiatric disorder in the immediate family, frequently depressive or psychotic in nature. One in twenty will own to a respiratory disorder, asthma being the most frequent. There is a representation of the less frequent problems, epilepsy, diabetes, Hodgkins, haemophilia etc. etc. Indeed one noticeable feature which increases year by year is the number of physically handicapped students coming forward to University. These present their own particular problems, probably more so for the Institution, in learning techniques and stresses although their academic achievement is very high indeed. Thus a blind student may need a team of up to twenty readers to cover the volume they are expected to cope with and the hearing-impaired may require review of the amplifying equipment to which they have access, and use. An appreciation of, and an interest in the communication and mobility problems of handicapped youngsters is essential clinical experience.

CONFIDENTIALITY

In several well structured projects, confidentiality emerged as the top priority a student expects of his medical services; not only is there a very real fear of information being passed on to or added to "files" held by college, but there is the long-standing suspicion that the family doctor is a confidant of the parents - hence why few willingly will seek help through generally accepted channels.

THE OCCUPATIONAL HAZARDS OF BEING A STUDENT

The university

The university is frequently blamed for being the cause of the difficulties but seldom really is, although these bodies tend to be very reticent at disclosing or even looking at the kind of impact they have on these young persons who come forward year by year. Suffice to say that the place merely sets the stage on which each student will act out his "play" which he brings with him from the home environment. It is not surprising that some of the "staff extras", who find themselves involved in these happenings are a bit confused and bewildered. Some universities are 24-hour-a-day 7-days-a-week experiences which are very difficult to get away from for a break, and where the pace can be many times faster than that of home.

The training

Each student brings with him the kind of training, or lack of it, from his home and school, the attitudes, the feelings, the unfinished business. Sometimes selection of university has been very considerably influenced by the VI Form ambitions of the school; for some this may be a form of persuasion for performance at a higher level than their abilities can cope with.

Other people

For the first time in their lives they will come across an "academic" whose selection was not based on teaching ability or interest in the pupil, but on scholarly and research prowess. Sometimes this remote disinterest can be seen as cold and excluding. The Professor, as Head of Department, can be quite a different person from the Headmaster or Father at home. The student will meet staff at all levels, not just academic, but technical, secretarial and domestic strangers in a much larger institution than he has ever been used to, the numbers may be as high as 20 000, no wonder a few ill-equipped will pack their bags and return home within a few hours or days, overwhelmed by anxiety and loneliness.

The peer group

This is probably the most powerful force that operates on a student once he arrives at University - almost always chosen within hours of arrival; frequently out of the anxiety to share stresses with someone against the many. These friends will condition his behaviour, his habits and interests, his patterns of work and indeed may well influence the academic outcome. Surprisingly little is studied about this influence although some papers have emerged in the past from the United States of America.

Himself/herself

Just as the experience of university is an accelerated one, so too the need to experience the choices which life offers - some of the experimental behaviour is safe, e.g. organised or wider sport; more of it is fraught with dangers such as drug abuse, alcohol abuse - sexual immaturity, and motor traffic accidents. All generations have their experimental behaviour but none so much as the present, probably because of the almost epidemic spread of news and media experience from other countries and cultures.

Freedom

Since the Second World War and probably as a result of antithesis to all that war connotes, there has been a loosening of the inhibitions and structures on which our society is based. One feature has been the discouraging of boundaries where "normal" or "acceptable" behaviour is set and regulated, hence the difficulties the young person experiences in setting these limits for himself.

The decision to work or not.
The decision to get up or not.
The decision to sleep or not and with whom!
The decision to drink or not.
The decision to eat or not etc. (anorexia nervosa).

Small wonder that many may experience confusion and muddle at the apparent aimlessness of their experience and the indifference of others to their situation. In some ways the experience of university has become an initiation rite into society.

THE PROBLEM AREAS

It is sobering to reflect that as many as 20 000 students will drop out of higher education annually, an enormous waste of people and resources, but not least of all a disappointment and frustration for the young persons themselves and their families.

Academic

Three-fifths of problems present through this channel, usually accompanied by varying degrees of anxiety and unhappiness. About ten per cent of students, if asked, will admit stress immediately before or during examinations and discussion of the difficulty experienced may allow the development of a strategy of coping. For a few, ensuring a good night's rest with a simple hypnotic may suffice, for others a mild short-acting anxiolytic an hour before the paper will desensitise the almost phobic intensity of their anxiety. Whatever is done has to be "sold" to the student with the expenditure of time as being the most useful therapy. For a small number behaviour techniques may be appropriate and should be well within the grasp of most caring persons. Work and study problems, choice of course, changes of course, techniques of revision, selection of study material are all worth exploring and discussing. An understanding of the sine-curve relationship of efficiency related to anxiety (motivation) would enable useful suggestions to be made not only about the number of efficient hours of study but the way in which the other, equally important factors, such as sleep, food, fresh air activities and friendships can lead to a balanced life style developing. There is no doubt that the kind of organisation which a student requires at University can, for most, be quite different from that learnt and taught at school. Indeed Universities can be criticised for their failure to put this kind of learning exercise in a much higher priority on the academic plan. Anxiety is almost synonymous with being a student although we use words to soften the impact "motivation", "interest", "keenness" - for a small number this can be a persistent feeling which can be difficult to dissipate even with the best of psychotherapy or counselling support. Tranquillisers are to be avoided other than for very brief spells of a few days, if longer term medication is advised then small doses of imipramine or amitriptyline, say 10 mg thrice daily, can be used safely and with effect - the latter especially if there is an associated sleep problem.

Emotional

Between 10 and 20% of students will experience some form of emotional stress whilst at college, mostly of a mild anxiety and/or depressive nature; between one and three per cent with severe or psychotic disease where manic-depressive disorder or schizophrenic breakdown occur requiring referral. Behaviour problems are frequent, almost always maladaptive, i.e. failure to effect the change necessary to cope with the stresses thrown up by the University experience or withdrawal from these or the use of inappropriate ways of adjusting. Listening and counselling techniques are the most useful form of support.

It is useful to identify some groups who may experience varying degrees of difficulty and anxiety:

147

i.   The confused - muddled - overwhelmed.
ii. Anorexia nervosa - bulimia - eating disorders, all exist and in considerable and increasing numbers.
iii. Vulnerable groups - the first child or only child in family. The child from the family where there has been loss of a parent - between 1/10 and 1/5. The handicapped young person, and the lonely and solitary ("schizoid").
iv. The suicide risk - overdoses are not infrequently experienced and can be reduced by a deliberately "open-door" policy for psychological problems and by encouraging student "samaritan" organisations and staff awareness.

Psycho-sexual

Late adolescence is a time for changing attitudes and experimenting behaviour, perhaps more in the sexual area than anywhere else; drives which reach their peak at this age are expressed in relating patterns. About 20% of female students arrive already established on the contraceptive pill and this figure rises to about 65% by the end of final year; in 80% the relationship is with a steady boyfriend. Thus the physician needs to constantly update not only his practice but his attitudes and perceptions.

i.   **Maturational questions** - advice-seeking on "normal" sexual behaviour, patterns of response and consequences. Checking out parental-adult attitudes and responses. Somehow seeking to interpret to the Institution the needs of this group in a way which can be acceptable and within a framework which fulfills the responsibility of education. Sometimes a request for contraception will precede a deeper worry and conflict.
ii. **Pregnancy counselling** both during and after, together with effective and anonymous pregnancy testing. In a population with a high proportion of immature female students it is not unusual for three out of four pregnancy tests to be reported negative; therefore assumptions of the pregnant state can set any counselling help at nought unless confirmed and tests should be repeated if any doubt persists. Unfortunately there are many reports of inaccurate results from do-it-yourself kits with disastrous consequences.
iii. **Termination of pregnancy counselling** with encouraging early seeking of help and referral - follow-up is essential in avoiding long-term sequelae (see also Chapter 17).
iv. **Sexually transmitted diseases.** Frequently a concealed approach covers a real fear where contact may be minimal or even absent. Literature and information is easily made available through local branches of Family Planning Clinics although in the present state of knowledge about AIDS opinions are yet unprepared as to the most appropriate advice to give.

Accidents

The commonest cause of death in the age group 15-25 is an accident - six out of seven a motor traffic accident. Up to 75% of students will play organised and competitive sport so sporting and ortho-paedic injuries form about one third of all medical morbidity. The skilful physician will remember that to advise rest and stop all activities is almost impossible in this group - ways of enabling classes to be taken, practicals to be produced and examinations to be sat require careful co-operation with the tutors, lecturers, and examinations department staff - they will frequently suggest ways of circumventing problems. A considerable advantage accrues in en-couraging training in basic first aid at all levels, the emergence of an attitude of safety awareness may prevent many accidents.

Drug abuse

Three questions which must always be asked in   Student Health Services:

a. When were you last abroad?
b. With whom did you last sleep?
c. What drugs have you taken?

As one in four of all young people have access to drugs of abuse if they want them, a high index of suspicion is vital in trying to understand how some students present their problems, recalling that the commonest source of drugs is the medicine cabinet at home and not as is popularly thought the illicit imported drugs. More damage is caused by substances much closer to home and easily available.

i. **Coffee** - in the mistaken belief that drinking a lot of coffee will improve energy and concentration and maintain work rates, quantities in excess of four cups "instant" daily can cause paradoxical depression with all the symptoms of that disorder and consequences. A small number may develop quite acute anxiety states but they usually know this and avoid anyway.

ii. **Alcohol** - causes more problems on the campus than all other forms of drug abuse behaviour put together and the incidence of both acute and chronic alcoholism in this age group has risen dramatically in the past twelve years. There are consequences with respect to accidents, work and behaviour. A vigorous and positive helping attitude is needed by all the caring services if a young alcoholic is to be prevented from becoming an old one. David Ennals' phrase "everyone likes a drink - nobody likes a drunk" should be etched across every hospital corridor and common room!

iii. **Tobacco** - Few now can doubt the dangers of smoking induced lung cancer and related disorders, yet far too few doctors posi-tively educate their young patients about ceasing their habit or never taking it up. The growth of no smoking areas indicates the desire of most to produce results and could easily and effectively be extended.

iv. **Drugs** - At any given moment it is estimated, in Britain, that half a million young people are experimenting with drugs; most will start at about the age of 14 and stop by 17 years; few will go on beyond 22 years. Thus this problem is one seen mainly in the later years of school. In further education estimates of activity are not easy - perhaps 1% on so-called "hard drugs" and 10% on soft. At present, experience suggests cannabis as being the most frequently used and whilst this may induce a psychological craving there is no evidence that it is addictive. In the ways and strengths that it is used in Britain it is unlikely that this drug causes too many problems other than legal ones, it does however introduce and familiarise the taker to the "drug culture". Heroin, cocaine and other powerful drugs are less easily available but the figures suggest usage is increasing rapidly. Heroin users in Britain are conservatively estimated at about 50 000. Help for the management of these problems should be sought from specialist units working in this field but unfortunately efforts are largely frustrated as the insight required for co-operation is either lacking or severely impaired.

If we were to pay rather more attention to the problems of smoking and alcohol disorders in young people than the more publicised but miniscule numbers on drugs, there could be a significant change.

Infectious mononucleosis (glandular fever)

No apologies are offered for selecting one infectious disease which is almost endemic in Institutes of Higher Education, particularly where a significant proportion of the students are resident and which is a cause of many an unnecessary student drop-out.

Treatment

i. In the early **acute stages**, especially if confirmed by blood findings, can be dramatic using prednisolone 100 mg on the first day and reducing rapidly over a week. This can eliminate most if not all the physical symptoms.

ii. **Post-viral debility** - often referred to as post-viral depression or post-viral exhaustion syndrome. This is found with many viruses, though in about 1 in 10 mononucleosis cases, characterised by excessive fatigue and in some cases hypersomnia together with the features of depression - disturbance of mood, difficulty in concentration, loss of interest, disturbances of appetite and vegetative symptoms. The appearance of these symptoms even in the presence of negative blood findings and in the absence of drug abuse, should suggest a possible post-viral disorder. They respond uniformly well to imipramine 10-25 mg

150

thrice daily over a prolonged period, sometimes many months. Again it is vital to "sell" this therapy and support for what can be an extended and debilitating exhaustion in a finely tuned academic.

iii. The type of hand-out which can be invaluable in the management of this virus illness can be found at the close of this section.

THE ROLE OF LISTENING IN TREATMENT

The management of the vulnerable student can be assisted and indeed made more satisfactory if the following factors, which profoundly affect his progress, can be elicited and **listened** to with skill and care. Sometimes if one of these factors is weak and can be strengthened, then, like a game of dominoes, the outcome for the student can be strikingly different:

Motivation

Perhaps the single most important factor in progress; not only motivation for being in further education, but sound personal reasons. Too frequently one associates difficulty with varieties of persuasion both directly by parental ambition or more subtly "well, all the people in the VI Form went to University", or, "I had a super teacher who went to ....". Promises of a better job soon lead to disillusionment.

Interest

In the subject of study; the place, the time, and the people both in authority and peer group. Strong interests in extra-curricular activities and events. Surprisingly a "good feeling" about the place is of prime significance.

Goal orientation

Not only for the goals to be achieved of entry to further education but the degree and class together with an immediate and long term future goal. These are significantly clear in 75% of students and is associated with success. This requires good organisation and dealing with the problems of transition thus transferring the training from school to college.

Home stability

Seems to play a highly significant role in the ease with which a student copes with studies and learning skills. Although one in ten discloses absence of a parent figure, this is nearer to one in five on interview response. Disturbed parental relationships repay careful exploration and sharing.

Health

Most students will average two medical consultations per academic year; where four or more episodes are recorded this frequently suggests an underlying stress situation, especially if for one recurrent item of illness. Masked depression will often present this way.

GLANDULAR FEVER

Nothing seems to strike more anxiety into the hearts of students (and staff!) than the mention of the dreaded "glandular fever" or to give it its correct title "infectious mononucleosis". This is a virus infection, one that is almost endemic in universities given their highly residential, almost closed community environment. For many years referred to as the "kissing disease" as it can be transmitted, but only directly, by this behaviour and also by coughing and sneezing.

Like all viruses it causes a "flu" like illness which may be brief lasting 2 or 3 days then an interval of up to three weeks later there develops a painful swollen throat together with fever. This can continue for seven to ten days during which the patient can feel quite ill with swollen tender glands, especially round the neck and jaw, though sometimes in the axilla and groin too. There may be a fleeting purplish rash especially marked if penicillin-type antibiotics are administered.

However, not everyone will develop these symptoms and signs indeed only ten out of a hundred students will ever feel sufficiently unwell to have to seek medical advice. If one studies groups of students at entry to university the incidence of previous infection is about 8%; when, however, one examines students leaving the institution about 88% have been exposed to the virus; most never even know they've had it!

The diagnosis can be made on careful clinical history and examination, together with an awareness of its prevalence in the community. Confirmation of the diagnosis by special blood investigations is a satisfying exercise but its value is largely academic, it neither assists the treatment nor the outcome.

The majority of patients settle with conservative measures such as brief bed rest, plenty of fluids, sponging to cool off if necessary, and the use of soluble aspirin both locally as a gargle for the painful throat and internally to help lower the temperature and ease any discomfort. Recovery is rapid and for most complete in two to six weeks and it is not necessary to isolate the patient nor is it of any value for them to go home! A few patients may run a longer course with recurrent episodes of fever and lethargy but if advised to rest when necessary then the minimum of interruption to normal life is sustained. Antibiotics are quite unnecessary as viruses do not respond to these - sometimes a concomitant throat infection may indicate this but usually patient "pressure" is the frequent reason for prescribing "something". Complications are fortunately rare and again respond rapidly to the appropriate measures.

There are some myths about glandular fever which are worth mentioning.

1. **You can't get it again** - like most viruses they can induce prolonged immunity, indeed the "illness" itself is the bodies immune response to the virus which has really departed before the person experiences symptoms, a form of "allergy" reaction. It does, however, have the capacity of sensitising the lymph gland system so that subsequent virus infections, e.g. the common cold, may simulate swollen glands etc.

2. **Your academic studies are affected - this is just not so.** Extensive studies have been carried out over several universities and many hundreds of students. There is no difference in academic outcome between either a control group or a group with glandular fever.

3. **Depression** - a very few patients will experience post-viral depression similar to that frequently experienced following influenza virus but prolonged. This is characterised mainly by a feeling of fatigue which varies from day to day together with some alterations in mood. There is a rapid response to the appropriate treatment although patients frequently soldier on for some time before seeking help.

In conclusion, it always surprises me how much distress this mild virus seems to cause psychologically both to students and staff. Certainly the difference if the patient is **not** told the diagnosis is remarkable, they shake it off like a dose of the "cold", indeed some physicians swear by this practice. I usually wait until they're better before telling - if I get the chance!

14

Dangerous patients

T G Tennent

QUICK REFERENCE GUIDE

INTRODUCTION

Our whole lives are surrounded by events which we may see as potentially dangerous: driving on the roads, flying in aeroplanes, living in a world of nuclear reactors, surrounded by people who smoke, eating foods from animals given hormones and antibiotics, and vegetables treated with insecticides - each has some level of risk and some level of potential harm but, pressure groups apart, we accept all or most of these as part of the daily pattern of life. All of us have within us too the ability to behave dangerously, so to that extent we are all "dangerous patients", but to become a dangerous patient one has to raise the probability of an action or activity, or develop a situation to a level which raises the probability of serious harm above a certain level (Walker, 1983). Many very similar situations, actions or activities which go above this level never result in anything remotely dangerous happening, sometimes because of the awareness of those dealing with the situation, but more often by dint of chance events and circumstances.

One of the difficulties in attempting to define the dangerous patient is that of either being over- or under-inclusive - which in the first instance could result in every patient-doctor interview being defined in terms of 'potential for dangerousness' content, and on the other, only identifying situations which to the least experienced would indicate danger. Again, another difficulty is that once a patient is defined as dangerous, sociological as well as medical actions and decision evolve, and once someone is deemed dangerous, the problems of their future management increase enormously. Once deemed dangerous, it is very difficult to remove this label.

By and large then, general practitioners should perhaps be more aware of the dangerousness of certain situations which difficult and disturbed patients can create or have created around them, rather than become part of an attritional process which is not easy to reverse. Although the following parts of this chapter concern people and diagnostic categories, it is hoped that they will be read with this important caveat in mind.

THE SORTING PROCESS

The assessment of dangerousness, then, involves an attempt to balance those factors in the individual which may be considered as instigators to aggression as opposed to those factors which may either positively or negatively relate to inhibitions against aggression. In making one's assessment, therefore, there are three areas which might be considered:

i. Factors immediately relating to the current behaviour of the patient.
ii. Environmental factors.
iii. Internal factors of specific characteristics of the patient.

Each of these areas should be considered in terms of their contribution to the balance between acting aggressively and controlling such actions.

Factors relating to the current behaviour of the patient:

a. Current behaviour of the patient

i. Is he overtly threatening violence or saying that he wants to kill someone?
ii. Is there a specific victim?
iii. If so, is the victim himself, someone close to his environment, or someone more remote?

155

iv. Does he have the means of harming someone (e.g. a weapon)?

v. Is he under the influence of "command" hallucinations?

b. **Environmental factors**

i. What are the patient's current domestic circumstances in terms of the support or the non-support that they give?

ii. What are the patient's current living situations in terms of supervision, lack of social space, adequacy of environment?

iii. What are the patient's current financial circumstances? What are the economic pressures upon him?

iv. Is he socially isolated or an involved member of the community?

v. Is he socially skilful or inadequate?

vi. What is his work situation and/or work prospects?

vii. What alternative environments etc., are available to him?

c. **Internal factors or specific characteristics of the patient**

i. Psychiatric illness: has he had a past history of psychiatric illness, and how did he respond and/or behave during these episodes?

ii. How does he relate to other people - as victims or as exploiters - within society? Does he see people as individuals, or merely as objects to be exploited? Does he see people as separate, unique individuals or merely as members of classes (e.g. blacks, snobs, etc.)?

iii. How does he relate to others? How does he relate to authority figures? How does he relate to those over whom he has authority?

iv. How does he relate to his family? Is there a history of conflict with either or both parents? What was his relationship to his siblings?

v. What degree of impulse control has he demonstrated in the past? What technique of control does he use? How does he respond to provocation? Has he behaved violently in the past? If so, how, and what, were the precipitating factors?

vi. Does he have any organic or possible organic features? (e.g. episodic dyscontrol).

vii. Is there any evidence of drug or alcohol abuse prior to or during the aggressive behaviours?

The assessment of dangerousness will involve trying to weigh the significance of these factors. It is impossible at present to quantify them in a way which allows appropriate predictions to be made. At present the most reliable predictor of future behaviour is probably past behaviour, and this, with the relative weights of the factors listed above, has to be taken into consideration in making an assessment.

Dangerous behaviour within the community is fortunately a relatively rare phenomenon. People who behave violently often do so within a context which allows their violent behaviour to be controlled at a level acceptable to those around them. Serious violent events occur most commonly between people who have some association or knowledge of each other. It is not usually a one-sided process and, indeed, research evidence suggests that the victims of violence may themselves have often been very violent or may have contributed very significantly to the violent event. It should be apparent, therefore, that violence between strangers is a relatively uncommon phenomenon, and violence in families or in social situations is much more common.

VIOLENCE IN THE COMMUNITY

People who behave violently in a more general sense have a higher probability of being psychologically disturbed than the rest of the normal population. The repeatedly aggressive offender, for example, in the majority fall into the category of psychopaths and their violence is merely one facet of multiple personal difficulties. A relatively high proportion of such people have an abnormal electroencephalograph and people who have a life-long history of repeated violent behaviour are worth looking at in terms of the possible existence of the **episodic dyscontrol syndrome**. The majority of persons showing this syndrome have a history of repeatedly responding violently to quite trivial stimuli, dating back to childhood or adolescence. Their outbursts of violence are sometimes preceded by an aura of some kind that may be followed by headache and drowsiness. A proportion (the size of the proportion depends on the sophistication of the examination) show evidence of minor neurological deficits; and multiple development anomalies are a frequent concomitant of this syndrome. It is thought to be due to some disorder within the limbic system, and carbamazepine appears to produce an improvement both in frequency and severity of the episodes.

That apart, the majority of violent episodes against non-specific individuals are the result of their presence in a situation in which someone is behaving violently or, more rarely, the fact that they represent the object of some "command" hallucinatory experience. "Command" hallucinations involving the infliction of serious physical violence on others should be assessed in terms of the duration of their presence; whether or not the individual has acted upon them before; the extent to which he is able to resist them and the extent to which he has been helped by medication. Even with hallucinatory experiences the check-list type questions mentioned previously help one in determining whether or not a patient is likely to act upon the hallucinatory commands that he is given.

FAMILY VIOLENCE

The practitioner is much more likely to be called upon to assess the potential dangerousness of the patients within their family situation. There are a number of situations that have been described: morbid jealousy, baby battering, wife battering and granny bashing.

Morbid jealousy (see also p.15)

This is sometimes the motive that drives a sufferer to kill the object of his possessiveness or sometimes the person he suspects of having a liaison with her. It has been labelled the "Othello syndrome". The sufferer becomes convinced that his partner is unfaithful and starts seeking proof that such activities are occurring. Thus he will examine articles of personal clothing and the bedclothes for evidence of sexual activity. He may look for signs of her involvement with other people; make searches through her handbag and drawers, letters, etc. He may follow her and spy upon her and, additionally, he may tax her with accusations of infidelity - often claiming that if she admits he will forgive and forget. When examined, the majority of this group exhibit no other signs of psychiatric illness. In particular, there are no other signs or symptoms of paranoid schizophrenia at the time of the examination. A small number, however, do subsequently develop such symptoms. The majority have some degree of sexual dysfunction and there is often other evidence of marital disharmony. A large proportion are found to have alcoholic problems in addition to their paranoid symptoms. This is a very difficult group with which to deal because the level of jealousy seems to vary from time to time, not necessarily related to the activities of the suspected partner. Marital therapy can be of assistance to such couples, but if the symptoms persist then probably the relationship is not redeemable and some form of dissolution of the situation should be attempted. It is not unknown for men to produce these symptoms in a number of successive relationships.

Baby battering

This emotive term was coined by Kempe (1962) as a deliberate attempt to arouse public concern. This poses one of society's most current public dilemmas: the dilemma resulting from the conflict between the right of the parent to have their child (and the evidence that parents are an important part of child development!) and the onus on the caring professions to protect children against their parents. The caring professions are now much more aware of the problem of the abused child, but often the problem of when it is safe to return a battered child to its family remains a difficult one. As will be apparent from the factors which we considered in assessing the likely potential for violence in any situation, these can change dramatically from time to time, and whereas it may be safe at a particular moment to return a child to its parents, constant monitoring is required to assess any change in circumstances that may upset the delicate balance between the exhibition of violence and its control.

While baby battering is not the exclusive prerequisite of any single personality profile or relationship constellation, most studies show that almost ninety per cent of battering parents have many of the following characteristics:

1. A history of violence and/or neglect in their own childhood
2. They have broken away from the parental home at an early age
3. They tend to have their first child earlier than the population in general
4. In about one-third of cases the child is illegitimate
5. They tend to select a mate of similar background and personality
6. They are socially isolated
7. They have violent outbursts of temper
8. They have unrealistic expectations regarding their child's behaviour
9. They have a history of mental illness such as depression or anxiety.

The more of these factors which are present, the higher the risk to the child. There is a small percentage of child-abusers who fall into one of the following four sub-groups:

a. Psychotic parents suffering from some form of delusional illness in which the child is incorporated.
b. The parents, although not showing other evidence of a psychosis, hold extreme beliefs in regard to child-rearing, perhaps in a pseudo-religious setting.
c. Cold, affectionless, sadistic psychopaths who self-righteously impose impossible disciplines on their children, punishing them severely for the slightest infractions.
d. Explosive, violent psychopaths with very little self-control, where the most minor frustrations result in violence which is totally disproportionate to the circumstances.

Parents who fall into any one of these four sub-groups cannot safely be left in charge of their children. At the moment it seems that treatment is unlikely to be successful in any event, and the risk to the child is too high.

While in theory there may be many agencies available to help these families (and it must be remembered that although environmental factors may increase the stress on parents, battering of children is not confined to any one social class), parents seem to have difficulty in using the agencies available effectively. In part, this is due to the parents' own difficulty in trusting people, or their own lack of verbal skills. In quite a number of cases, however, one or other parent has drawn the attention of social agencies to the problem, albeit in an indirect way. There is a tendency for professionals to want to think well of their clients, despite evidence to the contrary. Decisions to remove a child are difficult, and should only be made after the fullest discussion with all the professionals involved and the parents themselves.

Kempe and Kempe (1978) have drawn up a check-list which may help in arriving at a decision. The more positive answers there are to the questions the greater the risk of repeated abuse and the greater the danger to the child.

1. Was the parent repeatedly beaten or deprived as a child?
2. Does the parent have a history of mental illness or criminal activity?
3. Has the parent been suspected of child abuse in the past?
4. Is the parent suffering from loss of self-esteem, social isolation or depression?
5. Is the parent experiencing multiple stress (recent divorce, marital discord, financial problems, housing difficulties, etc.)?
6. Does the parent have a violent temper?
7. Does the parent have rigid, unrealistic expectations of the child?
8. Does the parent punish the child harshly?
9. Does the parent see the child as difficult or provocative?
10. Does the parent reject the child?
11. Is the parent on drugs or using alcohol? (see also Chapter 18)

Wife battering

This is an extremely difficult subject as the degree of abuse that women are prepared to accept from their husbands as "normal behaviour" varies to an extent that wife battering tends to become defined in terms of a wife's tolerance rather than the actual behaviour. Research into battering husbands is obviously very difficult. Few are prepared to co-operate, except when in custody, and these are an unrepresentative sample. Gayford (1955) defined a battered woman as "a woman who has received deliberate, severe and repeated multiple physical injury from her marital partner". In forty-four per cent of the cases studied, the offences occurred regularly when the man was under the influence of alcohol. The wounds were usually inflicted with fists or by kicking, but in twenty per cent attempts had been made at manual strangulation. Almost half claimed that, on occasions, some form of weapon had been used. A quarter of the women had been battered by their partner before they began cohabiting. Eighty-five per cent had sexual intercourse prior to marriage and fifty per cent were pregnant when the relationship became permanent.

Almost half the women described their own childhood as unhappy, but this must be viewed with some doubt. Only sixty-five per cent were brought up by their own parents at the age of fifteen. In twenty-three per cent violence had been a feature of their own parents' relationship. Seventy per cent of the wives had been treated by their ggeneral practitioners for symptoms of depression

160

or anxiety. Forty-two per cent had made suicide attempts. Few had revealed to the doctor their husbands' violence. Questioning, therefore, about husbands' behaviour towards them is an important part of the interviewing process.

Various attempts have been made to categorise the sorts of men and sorts of relationship that lead to wife-battering situations. Faulk (1974) published a report on twenty-three men who were remanded in custody for serious assaults on their wives. This group could be divided into those over the age of forty and those under that age. The over-forties almost all showed evidence of serious psychiatric disorder, while in the younger age group about half had psychiatric disturbance, and most of these were personality or neurotic disorders. This group obviously represents the extreme end of the spectrum of battering husbands, and the findings may not apply to those who keep their violence within some kind of limit. Faulk categorised these men into five groups:

i. **Dependent-passive**: This type of man tried hard to please a demanding, querulous wife. The violence was explosive and followed a specific act by the victim.

ii. **Dependent-suspicious**: This group was similar to the morbidly jealous group described under this section in connection with murder, though in some cases the jealousy did not have the full delusion intensity but was pervading the relationship.

iii. **Violent and bullying**: These men used violence and threats to gain their ends in most aspects of their lives. This group also showed evidence of alcoholic problems.

iv. **Dominating husbands**: Often successful in other aspects of their lives, these men seemed to regard their wives as subordinates who must obey orders without question. Violence might be precipitated by trivial events which they regard as a threat to their own authority.

v. **Normal stable and affectionate husbands**: In this group the violence occurred only at times of mental illness, characteristically during a depressive episode.

Granny bashing

It is difficult to estimate how many old people are the victims of deliberate injury inflicted by relatives or other people who are entrusted with their care. Old people tend to bruise easily, and ordinary gripping of their arm when helping them to stand or walk can produce bruising. Pushes or slaps can give rise to much more serious injury in an old person than a similar assault on a younger person. Violence towards aged relatives is said to be common in certain conditions or situations:

i. In situations where care has been given for a long period of time and where increasing disability finally produces too much stress on the caring relative.

ii. In families where considerable reluctance to take in the old person has been over-ruled by pressures from outside sources.

iii. Where the almost equally-aged spouse has to cope more or less alone with a demented partner.

There is great difficulty in assessing the account given by the old person of the incident. Some will deliberately deny any violence and claim that they fell or knocked into something. Others, however, will invent acts of violence as part of a paranoid illness arising from either a setting of depression, dementia or paraphrenia. The old person with severe memory impairment may be quite unable to remember the circumstances and may confabulate to cover the memory loss.

This, then, is a very difficult area for assessment, and the likelihood of such an event occurring should be assessed along the lines suggested earlier in this chapter regarding the various controls and dyscontrols in the particular circumstances relating to the event.

Where violence between aged spouses is alleged, the contribution of increasing organic factors must be weighed up and such comments must not be ignored.

FAMILIAL HOMICIDE

The "depressive" murderer

Depressed patients, particularly those who have personality difficulties, should be examined not just for the suicidal risk to themselves but for the homicidal risk to those around them. The individual who has nihilistic delusional ideas, fears that he may have infected other members of his family, concerns about the future course of world affairs, and the effects of world events on the future happiness of his family, should again be looked at in terms of the potential risk that he poses to his family. Again, it should be stressed that it is the balance of factors in the life of the individual that should be considered and not just the mental state of the patient. However, although the evidence that those who threaten to kill have no higher chance of killing others than themselves, all such statements should be taken seriously. In retrospective studies of people who commit homicide and then kill themselves, West (1965) found clear warnings of the impending tragedy had been given to others but had been unrecognized or disregarded. He emphasized the risk inherent in the case of potentially suicidal women who have small children (see also p.187).

Parents who kill their children

The majority of women who kill, kill their own children, whereas of the men who kill only about fifteen per cent kill their own children.

162

The majority of mothers who kill their children (excluding infanticide) are regarded as being psychotic at the time of the killing. This is supported to some extent by the great incidence of suicide or suicidal intents in women at the time of the killing. Only about one-third of the fathers who kill their children are regarded as having some form of psychotic illness.

There have been a number of attempts to classify the various types of child murder within the family on the basis of motivation or psychopathology. No attempt has been wholly satisfactory, but the following modified version of that suggested by Scott is probably as good as any.

1. **Mercy killing,** where the child is a real source of suffering or handicap, where there is little secondary gain for the parents.
2. **Psychotic killing,** where the killing is a direct result of some multiple psychotic illness.
3. **Killing as the end result of battery:** In these cases there will be evidence of repeated assaults.
4. **Killing in one explosive episode without previous evidence of battering:** In this type there are two sub-groups:

   a. Those cases in which the child itself acts as a stimulus in child battering by its behaviour, and
   b. Those cases in which the child is killed as a substitute for the person the killer actually felt murderous towards.

5. **Killing as part of sexual abuse or to silence a witness.** Though this is a theoretical possibility, it would seem to be almost unknown in parent/child murder,
6. **Deliberate killing of an inconvenient child**
   a. by assault or
   b. by neglect.

REFERENCES

1. Walker, N D (1983) Protecting people. In Hinton, J W (ed.) Dangerousness: Problems of Assessment and Prediction
2. West, D J (1965) Murder Followed by Suicide. Heinemann Educational, London
3. Scott, P D (1973) Fatal battered baby cases. Medicine Science and the Law, 13, 197-206
4. Kempe, C H (1962) The battered child syndrome. Journal of the American Medical Association, 181, 17-24
5. Kempe, C H and Kempe, R S (1978) Child Abuse. Fontana Books, London
6. Gayford, J J (1955) Wife battering. British Medical Journal, 1, 194-196
7. Faulk, M (1974) Men who assault their wives. Medicine Science and the Law, 14, 3, 180-183

15

Demented patients

Cyril Josephs

QUICK REFERENCE GUIDE

DEMENTIA

Dementia is a state of impaired cerebral function which is usually irreversible and due to brain cell damage. It is one of the forms of brain failure: the brain in dementia contains significantly fewer than normal brain cells.

Dementia is not a diagnosis but a syndrome for which a cause should be sought in case it be remediable.

Any experience of any nature is received by and makes an impression on the cerebral cortical cells. The number of cortical (grey) cells involved depends on the importance of the experience. The greater the number, the more lasting will be the experience and the greater the power of recall. Thus it can be seen that loss of grey cells impairs recall: memory is therefore imperfect and variable in dementia.

A useful analogy is that of the newspaper photograph. This is made up of many dots and the more dots there are per square inch of paper the clearer the picture. Reduction in the number of dots means they are more widely spaced, with blank spaces between which, if large enough, will eventually render the picture unrecognisable.

When functioning brain cells diminish in number, newer experiences are less likely to create a clear impression. Experiences in the distant past have been recorded and stored at a time when brain cells were adequate in number and are more likely to be capable of recall.

This description is probably grossly oversimplified but nevertheless is a useful hypothesis to remind us of the prominent feature of memory loss as it occurs in dementia. The demented patient tends to have marked loss of **recent** memory; he may retain distant memory to a variable degree.

Like all living cells, brain cells have a life span and it has been postulated that over the age of 20 years about 10 000 neurones die daily never to be replaced. It is somewhat reassuring to learn that the normal adult has sufficient reserve to cope with these losses throughout his lifespan. When a pathological state causes brain cells to die at a grossly excessive rate, dementia ensues.

Incidence

It is probable that ten per cent of people over 70 years of age suffer from intellectual impairment. About twenty per cent of those over 80 years have a significant degree of brain failure. Brain failure is the commonest cause of confusion in the elderly. (To strike an optimistic note, which is always desirable, those who fear that increasing age always produces increasing senility can be reassured that four out of five people over 80 years will **retain** their intellectual ability.)

CAUSES OF DEMENTIA

Alzheimer's disease is the commonest type of dementia, probably accounting for about 70% of cases. **Multi-infarct dementia** accounts for some 20% of cases. The remainder comprise dementia from various causes including subdural haematoma, intracranial tumour, vitamin B_{12} deficiency, neurosyphilis, alcoholism and normal pressure hydrocephalus. This latter group, although only accounting for some 10% of cases, is important in that the cause may be eminently treatable and full recovery possible. The longer the dementia has existed the less is the chance of recovery, so diagnosis as soon as possible is essential.

Multiple causes sometimes coexist. Thus it is not uncommon for someone with Alzheimer's disease to suffer multiple cerebral infarcts, compounding the problem.

Clinical picture

1. Alzheimer's disease

Stage 1 - Gradually increasing memory impairment and intellectual failure. Memory loss is mainly for recent events. At this stage there may well remain enough insight for the patient to be aware of his shortcomings and to suffer consequent depression and feelings of unworthiness and inadequacy. Delusions sometimes occur, particularly directed against those concerned with the patient's welfare.

Stage 2 - Tendency to wander aimlessly by day and night. Aggressiveness and increasing disorientation. Increasing neglect of personal hygiene and clumsiness in handling food. Insufficient awareness of common hazards can render fires, cookers and electrical equipment dangerous. Supervision becomes increasingly necessary.

Stage 3 - Profound memory loss both for recent and distant events. Confabulation is common and identities of well-known people and objects become hazy. Irritability, aggression, insomnia and incontinence add considerably to the problem of management.

Stage 4 - Complete disorientation, considerable helplessness, immobility, muscular weakness, loss of weight and appetite. Aphasia, apraxia and agnosia. Purposeless and repetitive movements. Exhausting outbursts of screaming and shouting. Total care is required.

The disease may last several years and only in the later stages are weakness and general deterioration of such a degree that the patient succumbs to infection or injury.

2. Multi-infarct dementia

Essentially the same clinical picture but the distinguishing feature is the episodic course with periods of relative stability alternating with those of sudden deterioration (stepwise deterioration).

3. The remaining mixed group

Will manifest signs and symptoms which vary according to the cause. On the whole the onset is more rapid, sometimes even sudden and comparison between the state before and after the dementia is more practicable.

DIAGNOSIS

The patient with dementia typically presents as an apathetic, humourless person with loss of recent memory and more or less preservation of distant memory. Sometimes he is the opposite of humourless: he laughs and smiles quite inappropriately and illogically. He has difficulty coping with simple, everyday tasks such as dressing: there is a tendency to lose familiar possessions: motivation is lacking and he performs inconsequential activities.

The patient can rarely give any logical history but when this is forthcoming from relatives and friends it can be invaluable, especially as regards the onset and progression of the condition. A dispassionate view from a spouse or near relative is very useful, but it is important to realise that close relatives are often unaware of, or reluctant to admit to the intellectual deterioration of someone dear to them. In the early stages of dementia the patient can often reply correctly to quite searching questions when prompted by a relative. Thus when the doctor asks the patient where he lives he may get an incorrect answer whereas the spouse promptly gets a correct reply when the question is asked in a leading way, e.g. "You know you live at so-and-so".

An Abbreviated Mental Test (AMT)

This is a questionnaire of ten questions. It is widely used, takes only a few minutes to work through and is a useful method of obtaining a relatively simple objective record of a patient's intellectual status. It may later be useful as a baseline for comparison and can itself give a clue as to the presence or absence of brain failure. Due regard must be given to the limitations of the test. Thus acute illness, intoxication, nervousness, deafness, depression or dysphasia can give a falsely lowered result. With a little practice the value of such testing increases.

An Abbreviated Mental Test (AMT)

1. How old are you?
2. Can you guess, without looking at the clock, what the time is to the nearest hour?
3. Give the patient a fictitious address to remember (e.g. 42 West Street). Ask him to repeat it to ensure that it has been heard correctly. At the end of the test ask the patient what the address was.
4. What year is it?
5. Where do you live?
6. Who is this? (Check the ability to recognise two people, for example the doctor and a nurse)
7. When were you born? (Day and month are sufficient)
8. When did the Great War (1st World War) start? (Or the last war if you think it more appropriate)
9. Name the present King or Queen (or Prime Minister)
10. Count backwards from twenty to one.

One mark is given for each correct answer: no mark for an incorrect reply. A total score of less than 7 is highly in favour of brain failure.

This simple questionnaire produces results which compare favourably with those produced by a longer questionnaire. The few false negative results which emerge can usually be eliminated by repeating the questions at a later date. A non-demented person will often memorise the questions and his answers: a demented person will not.

The questions can be inserted into a general history taking and need not be sequential. However, if the patient seems to have sufficient insight to appreciate that the memory is dubious, there is nothing wrong with questioning formally, having first explained that it is a method of assessing the extent of memory loss.

CT scanning

Has revolutionised the diagnosis of dementia and the improved equipment and technique allow detection of quite small lesions (about 1.5 cm). However, CT scanning is not yet universally obtainable and elderly demented patients often receive low priority. Those patients with dementia of recent and fairly sudden origin should certainly be scanned as subdural haematoma is not uncommon and can follow trivial injury which may have occurred unnoticed.

Blood tests, skull X-rays and lumbar puncture have their place in diagnosis, especially in the search for a cause which may be remediable. But enthusiasm for investigation must be tempered with caution and a degree of scepticism. Investigations which are non-invasive, harmless and not too uncomfortable are one thing: those which are highly unpleasant and possibly dangerous must be thoroughly justifiable. An example of the latter is lumbar puncture: it can be dangerous and difficult in a demented person and is only occasionally justified.

Normal pressure hydrocephalus is rare and presents with the classic triad of mental confusion, incontinence and spastic paraparesis with abnormal gait. The course is relatively rapid and although surgical provision of a CSF shunt can produce dramatic improvement, the procedure is hazardous and has an appreciable morbidity. On the whole, results have not lived up to expectations.

Benign forgetfulness

Occasional and temporary inability to recall names or relatively unimportant past events is a common experience in people over 60. The patient is fully aware of his lapse, has no other cognitive impairment, will often apologise for his forgetfulness and can be assured he is not becoming demented.

168

Intracranial tumour

Tumours can be very slow growing and can produce dementia of insidious progress. One has to be aware of the possibility and when suspicion is aroused, possibly by signs of increasing intracranial pressure, focal neurological signs or increasing drowsiness, further investigations (e.g. CT scan, EEG) are well worthwhile and can produce a happy outcome. Diagnosis can be difficult but success is more likely when careful physical examination is repeated at intervals when subtle changes in physical signs may emerge. A search for a primary lesion likely to give secondary cerebral deposits should always be made (e.g. carcinoma of the bronchus).

Depression

Depression is often mistaken for dementia and must be considered in every patient who is thought to be demented. The two conditions frequently coexist, especially in the early stages of dementia when the patient retains sufficient insight to appreciate his plight and to be depressed thereby.

With depressive pseudodementia there is often a personal or family history of depression. The patient readily admits to loss of memory yet may get a good score in a formal memory test (AMT). This does not occur with true dementia. The depressed patient tends to say "I can't remember": the demented patient tends to hazard a guess or justify his forgetfulness with a facile, incongruous or even ludicrous excuse. Depressed patients rarely conceal their depression and may be obviously distressed (see also Chapter 5).

Drugs

Sometimes drugs will produce a confused state which resembles dementia though the relatively sudden onset should arouse suspicion. Common offenders include barbiturates, hypotensives, benzhexol, tranquillisers, digitalis and alcohol.

When a confused and "demented" state has developed soon after prescribing a drug, it is a good maxim to blame the drug, to stop it and to observe the outcome.

Diogenes syndrome

Named after the Greek philosopher, Diogenes, who advocated a life of extreme simplicity and lived in a barrel, this fascinating condition must not be confused with dementia. The person has a complete disregard for social niceties. He lives by choice in a state of self-neglect and filth; stores rubbish (e.g. hundreds of old newspapers) and appears poverty-stricken, though he often has more than sufficient money and indeed may be wealthy. He is usually suspicious of everyone and may live the life of a recluse.

Whilst there may be psychotic signs and symptoms these are by no means the rule and one may be driven to the conclusion that the mode of living represents nothing more than an example of supreme eccentricity in someone of quite sound mind.

Parkinsonism and dementia

Parkinsonism is one of the commonest diseases of the central nervous system in old age and there seems to be a relatively high incidence of dementia associated with it. The link may be due to the fact that each is now thought to be due to a specific deficiency: Parkinsonism due to lack of cerebral dopamine, dementia due to lack of acetylcholine. Drugs are becoming more efficacious in relieving the signs of Parkinsonism, though there is not yet available one which is fully effective in halting the progression of the disease. As regards the drug treatment of dementia, results are so far disappointing, but research continues.

Thyroid function tests

A good case can be made for the routine testing of thyroid function in those who seem to be demented. (Perhaps it would be a worthwhile investigation in all patients over 65.) The yield in hypothyroidism may be small but since the test is non-invasive and inexpensive it seems worthwhile, as treatment is simple and the results often gratifying. The earlier in the disease that treatment is started, the more likelihood there is of an improvement in intellectual ability.

MANAGEMENT

1. Treatment of the cause

Always desirable but only feasible in a minority of cases. Nevertheless, it is always important to seek a cause, particularly if dementia is of recent and rapid development.

2. Supportive

A frank discussion with relatives encompassing the likely course of the condition and what can be expected of treatment in the widest sense is usually of great value. Relatives are able to voice their fears and guilt feelings when they realise that their changing affection towards a hitherto dear relative is far from unusual and, indeed, to be expected. They can better tolerate the stresses involved if they know that help is readily available, without hint of recrimination, whenever called for.

Diagnosing dementia does not signify immediate removal of the patient to some institution, and many patients will be better off in their own homes. Each patient must be assessed individually as each is different. Decision as to the type of care best suited will depend very much on how much help is readily available from local hospitals, social workers, health visitors and nurses. But of paramount importance is the help available from relatives and friends. Thus someone with mild dementia and no home support may need urgent admission simply because he wanders at night. At the other end of the scale, someone with marked dementia may be kept at home if excellent services are available. It must always be remembered that the carers need care. A demented patient requiring constant attention will rapidly exhaust the most devoted relative or spouse if periodic relief is not forthcoming.

3. **Specific drug treatment**

Since the advent of levodopa with its marked effect on the signs and symptoms of Parkinsonism, if not on its ultimate course, it is reasonable to imagine an effective treatment for dementia. Both are basically degenerative diseases.

Many drugs have been produced and more will continue to appear. So far, results are disappointing. However, since most of the drugs advocated seem to be harmless and relatively inexpensive, it is justifiable to try. This justification is particularly apt when one faces the fact that there is little else to offer. Those who condemn drugs out-of-hand are not usually against their being used on spouses or close relatives who are dementing.

Drugs said to enhance mental function fall mainly into two groups: the vasodilators, said to increase cerebral perfusion, and the cerebral activators which are said to increase cerebral metabolism. The former group include cyclandelate (Cyclospasmol) and isoxsuprine (Duvadilan). The latter group includes naftidrofuryl (Praxilene). Co-dergocrine mesylate (Hydergine) is said to reduce oedema of astrocytes. (It may cause troublesome bradycardia.) Oxpentifylline (Trental) is a vasodilator and reduces blood viscosity.

Each of these drugs has its devotees: there are many drugs available because we have not yet got the right one. It seems reasonable to try one or other for about 3 months after which it should be stopped if no improvement occurs.

Anecdote

I have one lady in her eighties under my care in a large Old Age Home, who was quite severely demented and insisted she always got to my clinic (held in the Home) via the Underground. After 3 months Hydergine, 4.5 mg at night, she showed some improvement in behaviour. After 6 months she suggested I was getting senile when I asked her how she found the Underground these days. She thought I ought to know she lived in the Home and had not travelled on the Underground for years. I have kept her on Hydergine and she has remained quite lucid and friendly despite increasing deafness. Whether the mental improvement is due to the drug must be conjectural, but the possibility that it is ensures that the drug will not be stopped, particularly as there have been no noticeable side-effects.

Symptomatic treatment

Whilst drugs play a relatively minor role in the treatment of dementia, they may be needed to control such troublesome manifestations as anxiety, agitation, restlessness, aggression and insomnia. It is humane to relieve distressing symptoms and is often justifiably expected by the relatives.

Drugs should be given in the smallest effective dose for the shortest time necessary, and in no way do they obviate the need for general supportive measures.

The **phenothiazines** are the most effective and well-tried drugs. There are many to chose from. All can have troublesome side-effects which include drowsiness, hypotension, hypothermia and extrapyramidal involuntary movements. Rarer complications include obstructive jaundice and agranulocytosis.

The **minor tranquillisers** can be of value when nervousness and mild agitation are troublesome: diazepam is probably the most popular.

Sedatives and hypnotics may be needed when night restlessness is a feature, which is common. It is advisable to use relatively short-acting drugs which have negligible hangover effect such as chlormethiazole (Heminevrin) or dichloralphenazone (Welldorm). There is no place for barbiturates in the treatment of dementia.

Antidepressants have an important, if limited, role to play in treating dementia. Depression frequently coexists, particularly in the early stages when enough insight may remain to allow the patient to appreciate his plight and to be depressed thereby. A trial of an antidepressant can be very rewarding, and may even disclose that the intellectual reserve is better than originally thought.

4. **Mental stimulation**

There seems little doubt that stimulating the demented brain can produce significant beneficial change, albeit to a small degree.

Recall systems, where the patient is encouraged to recall past events by means of old photographs, slides and discussion can create enthusiasm and stimulate motivation.

Reality orientation, usually supervised by trained workers, is a method of stimulating intellectual reserves in an attempt to make the patient more aware of his place in his family and in society; to bring him up-to-date with what is happening around him and where he fits in with his surroundings.

It may well be that any success following mental stimulation is due to making the best of what intellectual capacity remains in the brain. That stimulation is beneficial is probably due to the fact that the demented brain is rarely as severely damaged as appears at first examination. However, it is certain that any success from mental stimulation depends very much on the devotion, persistence and stamina of the providers. Stopping the therapy will often result in regression: stimulation is a long and continuing process.

PROGNOSIS

Dementia is a serious and frequently fatal condition. Those with Alzheimer's disease usually die within ten years; atherosclerotic dementia is usually fatal within two years. Individual cases vary widely from these figures. Demented patients are particularly susceptible to bronchopneumonia, strokes, fractures and other terminal catastrophes.

Diagnosing dementia should no longer imply a "switching off" by the doctor; a conviction that nothing can be done. The quality of life can usually be improved and custodial care should be required less often than hitherto, at least in the early stages of the condition.

CONCLUDING GUIDELINES

1. Always look for a possible cause for dementia. It may be treatable.
2. When confusion appears suddenly in a hitherto lucid old person, look for focal neurological signs. In their absence suspect some acute recent disease which is potentially reversible.
3. Sudden onset of "dementia" occurring soon after a change in medication has been made may well be due to the medication.
4. Resist the temptation to give sedatives without making a diagnosis and never do so without carrying out a physical examination.
5. The more clear-cut the cause of confusion, the less likely is there to be a coexistent dementia.
6. Drug therapy is relatively easy to initiate but other aspects of management are of greater importance.
7. Attention to defects of vision and hearing is of great importance.
8. Be ever aware of the constant strain on relatives who care for a demented patient.

SUMMARY

Dementia is a syndrome, not a diagnosis. Also called "brain failure". Several possible causes.

A. **Causes of dementia**

    1. **Alzheimer's disease** - Commonest cause - 70% of cases.
    2. **Multi-infarct dementia** - 20% of cases.
    3. **Remainder due to various causes** e.g.

        a. Subdural haematoma
        b. Intracranial tumour
        c. B_{12} deficiency
        d. Hypothyroidism
        e. Alcoholism
        f. Normal pressure hydrocephalus.

B. **Clinical features** - Gradual onset except when acute causal factor responsible e.g. subdural haematoma.

    1. Increasing loss of memory, particularly for recent events.
    2. Wandering by day and night.
    3. Aggressiveness, neglect of personal hygiene.
    4. **Late stages** - complete disorientation, immobility.
    Total care needed.

C. **End-results** of Alzheimer's and multi-infarct are similar: mode of **onset** differs.

    1. **Alzheimer's** - slowly and steadily progressive.
    2. **Multi-infarct** - step-wise deterioration - i.e deterioration process interrupted by periods of relative stability.

D. **Diagnosis**

    1. **AMT** to assess level of intellect.
    2. Blood counts.
    3. Thyroid function tests.
    4. Consider CT scan, EEG.

E. Consider **depression**. Important. Severe depression may be mistaken for dementia. Both may coexist: treating depression may improve intellectual status.

F. **Diogenes syndrome** - Usually **not** demented.

G. **Parkinsonism and dementia** often coexist.

174

H. **Management**

a. Direct attention at the **cause** where possible.
b. **Supportive**. Important to help the carers with hospital admission and attendance of nurse, health visitor, doctor. Day hospital.
c. **Drug treatment**. Limited possibilities.

   1. **Specific** drugs for dementia of doubtful effectiveness: vasodilators; cerebral activators.
   2. **Symptomatic** treatment. Try to control troublesome manifestations e.g. wandering, anxiety, insomnia.
      Useful -   a.   Phenothiazines
                  b.   Antidepressants
                  c.   Minor tranquillisers
                  d.   Sedatives and hypnotics

d. **Mental stimulation**. Important to make best use of what remains.
   1. Recall systems.
   2. Reality orientation.

I. **Prognosis -**   **Alzheimer's** - death within 10 years.
                     Multi-infarct - death within 2 years.

16

Problems arising after therapeutic abortion

Robina Thexton

INTRODUCTION

Studies carried out on women who have had a termination of pregnancy do not show significant numbers having a psychiatric breakdown. There is, however, widespread emotional disturbance, which causes patients to visit, or call out, their GP.

COMMON PRESENTING SYMPTOMS

- Depression (see also Chapter 5).
- Anxiety (see also Chapter 8).
- Sleeplessness.
- Nightmares.
- Confusion (see also Chapter 20).
- Panic attacks.
- Loss of libido.
- Acute marital distress.

TIMING OF PRESENTATION

Immediate - due to:

- Remorse.
- Guilt.
- Horror of the operative procedure.
- Feeling that the medical care was punitive.

These symptoms are exacerbated by physical factors of pain, bleeding, hormonal imbalance.

Later:

- At the time the baby would have been born.
- When other babies in the family are born.
- At the anniversary of the termination.
- At the date of the first birthday.
- In succeeding pregnancies.
- When later attempts to get pregnant have failed.

APPROACH TO THE INTERVIEW

It should be unstructured, the patient being encouraged to talk and the doctor listening sympathetically. The patient needs to share her feelings in a non-judgmental, caring situation.

FACTORS CAUSING SYMPTOMS

The doctor listens for the following points:

- How the patient experienced the practical arrangements surrounding the operation.
- How she felt she was treated by doctors and nurses.
- Is it a first abortion?
- Her age.
- Is she foreign born?
- Has she any live children?
- Is she single or married, divorced, widowed, living with parents or partner, or alone?
- Nature of her relationship with the putative father. Has he deserted her, or changed his mind about whether they should have kept the pregnancy?
- Sexual adjustment, before and after.
- Whether it was a first or second trimester abortion.
- Was it kept secret?
- Is there a religious affiliation?
- How much emotional support is she getting from those close to her?

- Was the request for termination her choice, or was there pressure from others?
- Has she had previous psychiatric disorder or suicidal thoughts?
- Is there a psychiatric history in her family of origin?
- In her childhood, was she separated from one or both parents?
- Does she seem unable to make a good ongoing relationship with her GP, or keep switching to different partners in the practice?
- Were possible alternatives to abortion discussed before?
- What is she feeling now - remorse, guilt, anger, grief?
- Was the ambivalence of her feelings acknowledged?
- Why did the pregnancy occur?

OVERT REASONS FOR THE UNWANTED PREGNANCY

- Ignorance of her body and the consequences of sexual intercourse.
- Ignorance of contraception, and where to get it.
- Having been raped or sexually abused.
- Ignorance that pregnancy can occur with genital contact only, without penetration.
- Inability to use contraception effectively, e.g.

    - Failure to take the pill according to instructions - forgetting it - omitting other precautions during illness - use with other drugs making it ineffective, especially antibiotics.
    - Use of spermicides on their own, without barrier.
    - Careless use of condoms.
    - Reliance on rhythm method.

- Failure of birth control even though used correctly:

    - Barrier method.
    - Intra-uterine device.
    - Failed vasectomy of partner.

COVERT REASONS FOR THE UNWANTED PREGNANCY

- Search for love and affection from parents, partner or a baby.
- To draw attention to herself because of other problems, conscious or unconscious.
- Because of unsatisfactory relationship with the partner (often breaking up).
- Attempt to hold on to the father.
- Excitement of risk-taking.
- To avoid court case, schooling, boredom.
- To obtain accommodation (in some regions).
- To prove fertility.
- To express adolescent defiance, where the struggle for independence is more important than the relationship with the partner.

178

If the doctor decides there is a covert reason, he aims to help the patient to work it out for herself. Therefore he must retain a neutral doctor/patient relationship. Expression of his own attitudes and opinions will make it difficult for the patient to understand her own. He should, however, be aware of his own feelings in an individual consultation - often a reflection of the patient's feelings.

CATEGORIES OF PATIENTS

It is useful to assess whether the patient is:

- Able to use the crisis of abortion to rethink her problems and conflicts, move forward in self-understanding, and live more happily afterwards.
- Able to use the experience as a maturing process following a long history of struggle in early life experiences, and to seek therapeutic counselling for a limited time.
- In need of continuing support because she has an emotionally deprived and inadequate personality, and had strong psychiatric reasons for the termination.

COUNSELLING

Post-abortion counselling consists of repetition of pre-abortion counselling, which may not have been adequate because of, e.g.

- Other options of adoption, fostering, not having been discussed, and the patient now regrets her decision.
- Inadequate warning of grief reaction and subsequent mourning.
- Incomplete understanding of conflicting feelings.

If the doctor avoids asking questions, the patient will reveal which of her feelings is most important to **her**. One way of getting at her feelings is to ask her to provide suggestions for the improvement of the abortion service.

The doctor must always elicit whether any psychiatric sequelae following the abortion are due to the abortion **per se** or to other factors in the patient's life, and should remember that a woman with a healthy personality never feels complete detachment from a conception anyway.

Success is when the patient can move forward to independence and avoid later problems of depression, chronic anxiety, psychosomatic disease, e.g. colitis, hypertension.

REPEATED ABORTIONS

If this is not the first abortion, an attempt must be made to understand the failure to control fertility when continuance of a pregnancy is always unacceptable. What makes **this** woman allow herself to get pregnant and then not wish to be the mother of a child? To be the latter, she needs enough basic security to be comfortable with the dependency of childbirth, and to expect continuing caring from others. She will not have this security if her own experience of mothering when she herself was an infant, was inadequate or inappropriate. A mother who could not give enough affection to her baby daughter may have damaged the ability of the grown woman to sustain a deep human relationship with a man or a baby. Driven back to act out the lost and deficient primary maternal relationship, the daughter tries to be a mother herself, but has insufficient confidence to carry it through.

Another sort of mother smothers her child with possessive love. Because she is unsure of herself as a feminine woman, she cannot separate from her daughter, through whom she hopes to live again, so that her immature daughter is not free of her mother physically, socially or emotionally. The unwanted pregnancy becomes a vehicle for the restorative and reparative wishes as well as the destructive ones, but the latter win. The mourning is over the loss of satisfaction of the woman's real needs and wishes. Referral for psychotherapy is often the only way forward for such women.

17

Puerperal emergencies

Ian F Brockington

QUICK REFERENCE GUIDE

ACUTE MENTAL ILLNESS IN THE MOTHER

Puerperal psychosis

Diagnosis: "Puerperal" or "postpartum" psychosis is the name given to an acute onset of severe mental illness in the first few days after childbirth. Typically these mothers are stable (both in personality and social circumstances) and in sound mental health at the time of delivery, though there may be a history of mental illness in the family and about one fifth have suffered a previous breakdown with full recovery. The condition is rare, complicating less than 1:1000 pregnancies, i.e. each practitioner can expect to see only one case in a lifetime of general medical practice. It is more common after the first pregnancy. It begins within 2-3 weeks of delivery, usually during the first week.

    The symptoms may be of a typical mania (overactivity, grandiosity, loss of reserve, euphoria or irritability), acute schizophrenia (bizarre delusions, auditory hallucinations and passivity experiences) or a mixture of the two (schizoaffective mania) and there is often an element of confusion. There is no malevolence towards the infant, but he is at risk from accidental injury (e.g. one mother nearly choked her infant trying to feed it with an apple). The differential diagnosis is from established psychotic illness, especially chronic paranoid schizophrenia present throughout pregnancy.

A 28-year-old woman, with a calm and reasonable personality, became very irritable 3 days after the birth of her first child. At the slightest opposition she would swear and start smashing crockery. When the doctor arrived, she dashed into the street, shouting and hammering on the neighbours' doors. A dangerous situation developed, and the baby had to be kept out of the way. She was eventually escorted to an ambulance and taken to hospital. Her mood was elated and she required very little sleep. She made a full recovery in 6 weeks.

Action:
1. The patient needs sedation with phenothiazines.
2. An urgent consultation with a psychiatrist should be obtained.
3. Hospital admission is usually necessary, either to an acute psychiatric ward without the baby, or to a psychiatric mother-and-baby unit. Compulsory admission under Section 2, 4 or even 135 may be required.
4. If the baby is not admitted, provision for his care, and the care of any other children must be made.
5. The family can be reassured that full recovery is expected in all cases.

Puerperal and postnatal depression

Diagnosis: Depression is quite common in the aftermath of childbirth. A wide spectrum of severity and clinical pictures is seen. Some are acute, with psychotic features, developing in hitherto normal women during the first 2-3 weeks; these may be a depressive form of puerperal psychosis. Others are mild and develop later, e.g. 6 weeks or 6 months after delivery. Others are chronic, starting during pregnancy, or associated with personality disorder and multiple social problems.

Surveys have shown that 15-20% of mothers develop postnatal depression; however some of these illnesses are brief, and many patients will not consult their general practitioner. The figure for prolonged depression, lasting 6 months or more, whether starting in pregnancy or after delivery, is between 5 and 10%. Thus each practice will have a number of cases each year (see also Chapter 5).

A 25-year-old woman presented 6 weeks after the birth of a baby girl. She was the wife of an executive, and was shy and diffident compared with her sociable and popular husband. She was distressed by his lack of support at the time of delivery. She became profoundly withdrawn, almost mute and was unsure whether she was still alive. She remained in this state for some months in spite of energetic treatment. Her husband denied any marital friction, but there was evidence of physical abuse. It eventually emerged that he was having an affair. When this came to light, the patient recovered and the marriage survived.

Action:
1. Chronic maternal depression is a neglected problem, and has serious effects on the family environment. There is a need for diagnosis in the first instance. Here the health visitor has an important role, but her visits cease after a few weeks, and the main responsibility rests with the family practitioner.
2. Many of these depressions are psychologically and/or socially determined and the predisposing factors must be identified and dealt with if possible. Combined assessment by doctor and social worker, health visitor or community psychiatric nurse (making a home visit) is useful.
3. Mild and brief depressions can be managed in primary care.
4. It is important to involve the husband in treatment. Social casework may also be necessary.
5. Severe and chronic or resistent patients should be referred for psychiatric treatment. A few will require admission (preferably with the baby), but this is disruptive to the family.

THREATS TO THE SAFETY OF THE NEWBORN

Incompetent mothering

Diagnosis: This usually occurs when the mother is mentally handicapped, or suffering from severe chronic mental illness (schizophrenia, alcoholism or drug abuse). It may also occur when the mother is immature, irresponsible and unsupported by mature adults.

Action:
1. The general practitioner and obstetric services should be aware of the existence of chronic mental illness or mental handicap during pregnancy. Midwives and health visitors should be alerted to the risk of neglect or accidental injury to the infant.
2. If the mother's behaviour gives cause for concern, the social services should be involved.
3. If mental illness is present, the mother should be referred to the psychiatric services.
4. A mother and baby home run by the social services or voluntary agencies is a useful resource providing shelter, supervision and an opportunity to learn maternal skills.

Irritable mothers

Diagnosis: Mothers come under great pressure during the first few weeks and months after delivery. They are often short of sleep, and this makes them more volatile. There may be great demands not only from the infant but other young children as well. They may be under considerable emotional tension, and may be unduly irritable. They may come to the surgery and complain that they are "at the end of their tether".

A 24-year-old mother presented with marked irritability 4 months after the birth of her baby. Her sleep was interrupted several times each night. In the surgery it was obvious that she was very fond of the baby, but she was labile in mood and exasperated with him. She was advised to satisfy herself that the baby was safe and comfortable, then let it cry so that it could learn a proper sleeping habit. She was greatly relieved by this advice.

A 21-year-old unmarried mother presented at the surgery with her 6-week-old baby. She had a history of antisocial behaviour, assault and parasuicide. Her boyfriend had absconded with their savings a few days before. Since then she had hardly any sleep. She was hitting the 3-year-old but appeared fond of the baby. She was persuaded to accept admission to hospital. With social casework and psychotherapy she soon settled down, and was discharged after 5 days.

Action:
1. In mild cases, the practitioner should intervene to ensure that the mother gets adequate rest. She may need counselling about leaving a crying baby to settle. She may need one or two nights under sedation while someone else looks after the family. Early in the puerperium a brief readmission to the maternity hospital may give her the support she needs.
2. It may be appropriate to consult with the health visitor or social worker.
3. In severe cases psychiatric referral for investigation of social circumstances and family dynamics is necessary.

Delayed maternal attachment

Diagnosis: The development of maternal feelings and of an emotional attachment to the child is not immediate and automatic in all or even most mothers. There is often a period of days and weeks in which the mother has not yet recovered from the ordeal of parturition, and the infant is difficult to manage. Maternal attachment probably develops as a result of the social interaction between mother and infant, to which the infant makes an important contribution. Delayed attachment is common when the pregnancy was unwanted, and is more frequent if delivery is complicated or if the infant is retarded, but it may also occur in favourable circumstances.

The frequency of attachment delay of at least 6 weeks is probably about 10%, but many mothers conceal their feelings because they are ashamed of them. It should be distinguished from the other disorders of mother infant relationship described below.

Action:
These mothers require explanation, reassurance and encouragement. Almost all will develop a normal attachment in the fullness of time.

Rejection of the baby

Diagnosis: This is a severe form of delayed attachment in which the mother hates her baby and wants to be rid of it. It probably complicates about 1% of pregnancies. It should be distinguished from depression with feelings of unworthiness in which the mother feels the baby would be better off with a different mother.

A 26-year-old mother gave birth to a boy after a planned pregnancy. 5 months later she was admitted with "depression" after slapping the child. She said, "I can't bear him; I don't want to know him". She insisted on his removal, and he was placed with his paternal grandparents. She remained depressed for nearly 3 years in spite of psychotherapy, marital therapy, in-patient admission, electroconvulsive therapy and several courses of drug treatment. Relationships within her family and with her in-laws were stormy. When the child was 3 years old, a clinical psychologist, working directly on the mother-child relationship, established a normal '"bond" within 3 months, and she recovered from her depression.

Action:
1. These patients need expert assessment by a psychiatrist.
2. The social services should be involved because the infant is at risk.
3. Joint admission of mother and baby may be beneficial.
4. Treatment is difficult, though not impossible. If it fails the baby will have to be placed elsewhere.

Obsessions of infanticide

Diagnosis: It is not uncommon for scrupulous and decent mothers to experience distressing impulses to harm their babies. These are obsessional phenomena and do not put the baby at risk, though they may lead to a mother avoiding contact with her baby and feeling distressed in its presence.

Action:

1. Most cases will not come to the attention of a doctor because mothers conceal such shameful impulses.
2. When these impulses are severe and troublesome, it would be wise to refer the mother to a psychiatrist because of the differential diagnosis from more severe conditions.

Child abuse

Diagnosis: The baby is injured by blows, shaking, scalding or burning. Alternatively the baby is deliberately starved or neglected. The setting for this is usually personality disorder, lack of social support and mental handicap rather than rejection of the baby. The diagnosis depends on actual harm to the infant. This is rare (1:1000).

> A 25-year-old unmarried mother, who had 4 children by different fathers (two already in care), lost her temper with her 2 little girls because they made a mess on the floor with their jigsaw puzzle. She burnt the legs of her 3-year-old against an electric fire. In the resulting enquiry it emerged that the mother had given trouble from an early age, and been involved in prostitution. The injured child was removed into foster care. The patient was given regular supportive psychotherapy for 2 years and appeared to have a good relationship with her remaining child.

Action:

1. The practitioner should be aware of the risk in certain groups of mothers; midwives and health visitors should be alert.
2. If, because of the background circumstances or the attitude of the mother, you think that there is a **risk** of neglect or injury, the social services should be alerted. It may be wise to refer the family to a child psychiatrist. Prophylactic referral to the National Society for the Prevention of Cruelty to Children may also be useful.
3. When actual abuse is **suspected**, a paediatrician should be involved. He will bring in other members of a specialist team, including the police. The social services must be involved, and they will call a case conference to hear all the evidence and make the decision about the future care of the infant and other children.
4. If the child is not removed from the mother, he should be supervised vigilantly, with daily inspection (e.g. at a nursery); meanwhile the mother and family require skilled psychotherapy.

The law: acting in an emergency: If there is reason to suspect that a child is being assaulted, neglected or ill-treated, application can be made to a Justice of the Peace for a warrant authorizing a constable to Enter and Search, and if necessary remove the child to a

Place of Safety. The police, acting on the authority of the Station Officer (in lieu of a magistrate), can take the child to a Place of Safety for 8 days (Section 40 of the Children & Young Persons Act, 1933). A Justice of the Peace can detain the child for 28 days (Section 28 of the Children & Young Persons Act, 1969).

Care orders: If the Social Services have reason to believe that a child's proper development is being avoidably prevented or neglected, or his health impaired or neglected, or he is being illtreated, he can be received into voluntary care with parental agreement (or without their objection); the parent then has the right to take the child back. If the parents do not agree, the Social Services can make an application to a Magistrate's Court for an Interim Care Order, which gives the Local Authority the rights and duties of parents (Section 2 of the Children & Young Persons Act, 1969).

Infanticide

Diagnosis: This is excessively rare and is mentioned only for completeness. It occurs in a variety of settings.

Action: If a mother has killed her baby, she needs immediate admission to hospital for assessment and treatment. The risk of suicide is high. The police are informed. Trial and prolonged treatment and rehabilitation are necessary (see also p.162).

18

Emergencies arising from the non-medical consumption of drugs

Martin Mitcheson

DEFINITIONS

The word "drugs" in this section refers to those drugs acting on the central nervous system, deliberately consumed for their psychic effects other than in the course of bona fide medical practice. Nicotine, however, will not be considered. Alcohol is by far the commonest drug consumed in this country and frequently consumed in combination with, or as a substitute for, the drugs described below. This chapter is primarily concerned with emergencies and is not concerned with the psychological side-effects of drugs prescribed for somatic disorders, nor the overdose effects of substances consumed for deliberate self-harm, other than accidental or deliberate overdose resulting from consumption of psychoactive drugs as defined above, and does not attempt to provide a general over-view of many questions regarding the long-term risk of drug taking, or to discuss the contentious social aspects of control and prevention or the appropriateness or otherwise of long-term maintenance prescribing. Suggestions for further reading are included under references.

MEDICAL EMERGENCIES FROM MISUSE OF PSYCHOACTIVE DRUGS ARE:

Overdose; accidental or deliberate;

Acute adverse reactions, including intoxication produced by sedative tranquillisers including volatile inhalants, panic reactions resulting from consumption of a variety of drugs, drug-induced paranoid states;

Withdrawal illness from sedative tranquilliser group;

Medical and surgical complications associated with drug misuse.

Other situations need to be considered. Families may, however, construe any non-medical use of drugs by one of their members as an emergency. Persons with responsibility for young people, such as residential home staff, or school teachers, may react similarly. Consumers may regard a request for supplies of stimulants or opiates as an emergency when their usual sources of supply are interrupted.

Most physicians would agree that any use of drugs by a pregnant woman constitutes a need for an urgent consultation on behalf of the foetus.

CLASSIFICATION:

Before considering the four main emergencies in detail the practitioner requires a framework within which to assess the urgency and appropriate response. Drug use and misuse can be classified in many ways, but for this chapter, in addition to the nature of the emergency itself two classifications are most relevant in responding to it.

1. **Classification by pharmacological action:**
(The examples in each category are not comprehensive.)

i. **Sedative Tranquillisers:**
Alcohol;
Barbiturates, e.g. amylobarbitone, Tuinal, Nembutal, pheno-barbitone;
Benzodiazepines, e.g. diazepam, chlordiazepoxide;
Other sedatives, e.g. meprobamate, chlormethiazole, meth-aqualone, glutethimide, chloral;
Volatile inhalants, e.g. organic glue solvents (especially toluene), butane, carbon tetrachloride, aerosol propellents.

ii. **Opioids:**
Natural and modified opiates, e.g. opium, morphine, codeine, heroin;
Synthetic opioids, e.g. methadone, pethidine, dextromoramide, dipipanone, buprenorphine.

iii. **Stimulants:**
Amphetamines, e.g. dexamphetamine; (popular proprietary pres-cription medications of amphetamines in combination with bar-biturates are no longer marketed in the United Kingdom.)
Amphetamine-like, e.g. methylphenidate, diethylproprion;
Cocaine;
Caffeine, e.g. coffee, tea, cola drinks.

iv. **Psychedelics** alternatively referred to as hallucinogenics or psychotomemetics;
Lysergide, psilocybine (mushrooms);
Dissociative anaesthetics, e.g. phencyclidine (PCP);
Cannabis, marihuana.

2. **Classification by style of use:**

This classification is of value in planning longer-term treatment and advising anxious families and professionals responsible for institu-tions. There are overlaps between these categories and intermediate cases.

Type One - intermittent consumption of drugs for psychic effect without development of tolerance or physical withdrawal illness. Not strictly drug dependence, but may be associated with overdose and adverse reactions.

Type Two - daily consumption of drugs singly or in combinations, often by injection, with the object of obtaining a psychic effect. Tolerance usually present. Withdrawal symptoms generally ex-perienced if daily use discontinued. Frequent substitution of alter-native drugs when drug of choice not available, e.g. purchase of over-the-counter codeine-containing cough mixtures or consumption of alcohol when illegal drugs in short supply. Use may be a subcultural activity.

Type Three - daily consumption, usually by mouth, of a stable dose. Only moderate tendency to increase dose if tolerance develops. Often drug taking initiated by medical prescribing and supply continued by prescription. Motivation to continue may be to control original symptoms for which drug prescribed, and/or to avoid withdrawal symptoms. Use tends to be solitary.

Except in emergencies Type One is not usually the concern of the medical profession. Type Two is often associated with social complications of drug use, and in the past it has certainly been acceptable British practice to consider moving a patient from uncontrolled Type Two consumption towards Type Three by authorising a medical prescription. This practice is the subject of debate and controversy.

MANAGEMENT OF OVERDOSES

The dividing line between an overdose and an adverse reaction is not necessarily clear cut. The term overdose here will refer to the direct toxic effect of excessive consumption upon vital functions. Adverse reactions will cover the direct behavioural consequences of excessive drug consumption.

Overdoses should usually be referred direct to hospital. Pending arrival of an ambulance, and during transit to hospital, it is essential to maintain vital functions and, in the case of opioid overdose, there is a specific antidote - naloxone - which should be included in every doctor's emergency kit. It is important to try and determine the nature and quantity of drugs consumed. Information should be obtained from associates, as well as from clinical examination of the patient. Containers of drugs should be requested for determination of contents and sent with the patient to hospital. Subsequently, information from the containers may enable referral to be made to supplying pharmacist and prescribing doctor.

Overdose of opioids

Diagnosis: Depressed respiration, pinpoint pupils and a relatively shallow coma are classical signs of opioid overdose. Severe respiratory depression may result in fixed dilated pupils.

Management: The immediate and usually effective treatment is the slow intravenous injection of naloxone in a dose of 0.4 mg. If a rapid improvement in the respiratory rate is not observed then it is strongly suggestive that either opioids are not the cause of overdose, or another drug has been taken in combination. Where the

191

overdose has been of a long-acting drug, such as methadone, continued observation is required, with repeated administration of naloxone as necessary. In the physically tolerant and dependent individual, naloxone will produce acute and distressing withdrawal symptoms resulting in extreme agitation, anguished demands for administration of an agonist opioid, which should possibly be given in small doses subject to careful observation. Positioning of the patient, in the semi-prone position where, if vomiting should occur, abdominal contents are not aspirated, is important. Experienced drug users occasionally develop a hypersensitive response to heroin with acute pulmonary oedema. It is not clear whether this is dose related. A mixed overdose is a common occurrence. It is unusual, though not impossible, for death to occur solely from opioid overdose. In the majority of Coroner's cases involving deaths associated with opioids reported in this country, sedative tranquillisers and especially alcohol have also been implicated, having a synergistic effect.

Sedative tranquilliser overdose and mixed overdose of central nervous system depressants

Diagnosis: Overdose is characterised by a depression of central nervous system, respiratory and cardiovascular functioning. The signs are similar to those of varying degrees of anaesthesia with progressive depression of consciousness, pain reflexes and muscular reflexes. Examination is also required, for evidence of trauma, possibly occasioned by ataxia resulting from drug consumption, and, if coma has been prolonged, for pulmonary complications of cardiac failure or infection.

Management: Patients suffering from sedative tranquilliser overdose would generally require transfer to hospital and continued observation, the exception being where the patient is rousable and may be able to walk to the surgery and facilities are available for close observation should the patient pass from state of intoxication towards coma.

If, but only if, the patient is only slightly intoxicated and is awake, then after the history has been taken and a physical examination carried out, vomiting may be induced through the use of syrup of ipecacuanha. No attempt should be made to induce vomiting in the patient who is semi-comatose or comatose because of the risk of aspiration of stomach contents. In the deeply comatose patient an endotracheal tube should be first introduced and then gastric lavage undertaken. Such procedures, of course, should normally be confined to a hospital based service. During transport to hospital the patient should be lain in the semi-prone position to reduce the risk of aspiration of vomit and an airway maintained. Mouth-to-mouth respiration or use of an ambu-respirator must be undertaken if respiration is depressed and cyanosis present. It should be noted that deaths have occurred amongst users of illegal drugs because of a fear that the police may be informed, resulting in prosecution of associates who might otherwise have arranged life-saving help. While this is a matter for individual ethical consideration, the management of the acute emergency is obviously facilitated by a guarantee of medical confidentiality. Barbiturate overdose is a declining problem because of the reduced availability of barbiturates associated with marked reduction in medical prescribing and the substitution of the safer benzodiazepines. Accidental overdose is paradoxically more likely to occur in the regular heavy user of barbiturates who has developed physical tolerance to the "desired" effects, but not to the respiratory depressive effect. The safety ratio between a dose required to produce sedation and/or euphoria, to the dose that produces respiratory depression, narrows as tolerance to the drug is acquired.

Overdose of volatile inhalants

In terms of useful medical intervention this is unlikely to produce an emergency because as with those volatile inhalants used for the induction of surgical anaesthesia the effect is generally reversed quite rapidly since the drug is eliminated naturally by respiration. Death can, however, occur if the consumer inhales the drug by placing their head inside a bag, or inhaling in small confined spaces such as cupboards. Death may also occur by acute vagal stimulation inducing cardiac arrhythmias when solvents are combined with an anxiety provoking situation. Asphyxiation may occur when the **relatively** safer glue solvents, such as toluene, are replaced by attempting to inhale pressurized butane or aerosol propellants, with the consequence that the gas may produce asphyxiation.

Management: of the patient with respiratory depression is to maintain an airway during recovery.

Stimulants

Diagnosis: Overdose is most likely to occur amongst athletes utilising these drugs to improve performance, or amongst persons attempting to smuggle large quantities of drugs by ingesting balloons or condoms which rupture in the intestine. The symptoms are those of over-stimulation and over-activity with cardiac arrhythmias, hyperthermia especially in athletes competing in hot weather conditions, hypertension, and occasionally convulsions. Concurrent use of monoamine oxidase inhibitors (e.g. parnate, phenelzine) dramatically increases the risk of hypertension and cerebral haemorrhage.

Management: Consists of rest; use of sedatives such as diazepam which may be given by intravenous injection if convulsions occur; ice packs for hyperthermia.

Psychedelic drugs

These seem to be relatively safe in overdose; see below for adverse reactions.

ACUTE ADVERSE REACTIONS, PANIC ATTACKS, INTOXICATION

Opioids

Opioids do not generally produce disturbing experiences, although not all individuals experience opioid consumption as euphoric. Vomiting frequently occurs in the inexperienced user, but is not generally experienced subjectively as distressing.

Sedative tranquillisers
(See Chapter 3)

The symptoms and management are as described for alcohol. It is worth noting that consumers may experience acute anxiety or fleeting hallucinatory experiences under the influence of these drugs, especially the volatile inhalants.

Psychedelics

This group of drugs can give rise to acute panic reactions, popularly referred to as a "bad trip". These can occur in relatively experienced users even after a number of pleasant experiences. They are most likely, however, to occur amongst novice consumers; those taking the drug in anxiety-provoking situations; older persons experimenting with an unusual experience, and perhaps particularly at risk if discovered in the course of an illegal activity; any consumer who unexpectedly encounters an unaccustomedly large dose. Adverse reactions are relatively uncommon with the relatively weak psychedelic drug cannabis, particularly when this is consumed with some care by inhalation; it is more likely to occur when cannabis is consumed by mouth with less control over the dose.

The predominant symptom and sign of an adverse reaction is acute anxiety which may be related to subjective perceptual disturbances, or to external anxiety provoking events. In a severe reaction the patient may experience true hallucinations, but is more likely to be experiencing distortions of real perceptions. The perceptual disturbances, often including synasthesia - a confusion of sensory modalities, whereby, for example, sounds are perceived as "seen", - may lead the patient to believe they are experiencing a serious psychiatric illness. The occurence of sympathomimetic effects with increased heart rate may lead to fears of imminent physical death.

194

Management of these acute reactions is first, second and third, reassurance. This requires caring for the patient in a situation with minimal sensory stimuli and reducing outside disturbances; reassurance, often repeated since short-term memory may well be affected, should relate the person's current psychic experience to the fact that they have consumed a drug. In fourth place to reassurance the use of tranquillisers may be considered, but this should only be necessary where it is not possible to organise reassurance in an appropriate environment such as may occur in the sort of large public gatherings where drugs may be consumed. Benzodiazepines are the drug of choice, e.g. diazepam 2-10 mg by mouth. Phenothiazines should be avoided both because they are less effective, and because the atropine-like effects may accentuate the effects of the dissociative anaesthetics if these are the causative agent. Psychiatric hospitalisation is very rarely necessary and should be avoided if at all possible because it is unlikely to be effective and may exacerbate the person's fear that they are indeed going mad, particularly when confronted with disturbed psychotic patients in an acute admission ward. Where the patient continues to experience perceptual disturbance and panic beyond a period of 24 hours, then consideration must be given to the likelihood of an underlying psychiatric illness. The incidence of acute adverse reactions to psychedelic drugs has probably been increased in the past by the publicity given to bad trips, because of an increased sophistication both amongst consumers who may take more sensible precautions, and amongst professionals working with drug users who have acquired the skills to manage adverse reactions by psychological reassurance.

Recurrence of adverse reactions, popularly known as "flashbacks", may occur, particularly when somebody has had a seriously disturbing psychological experience. They are probably a learnt response recalling a disturbing situation rather than any chemically mediated change of brain structure. Flashbacks are generally self-limiting, but may require administration of a small dose of a benzodiazepine tranquilliser. Reassurance and attendance to underlying anxieties are important.

Stimulants

Acute anxiety and over-activity can occur. Paranoid reactions are the principal serious adverse reaction to both amphetamines and cocaine. Individual dose response can vary widely. The acute paranoid episode is indistinguishable phenomenologically from acute paranoid schizophrenia.

Diagnosis depends upon a high index of suspicion with the immediate collection of a urine sample for subsequent confirmation.

Management: The disorder is generally self-limiting within a period of two or three days, if the person can be contained in a situation where access to drugs can be absolutely denied - this does not necessarily include most hospital wards or even prisons! Repeated urine testing, however, can explain the continuation of paranoid illness. Unless the patient is very disturbed, medication with major tranquillisers should be avoided since this may obscure the diagnosis and is unnecessary. Acute anxiety is best controlled by prescription of benzodiazepine minor tranquillisers.

DRUG WITHDRAWAL EMERGENCIES

Withdrawal from sedative tranquilliser group of drugs

Withdrawal from this group will be considered first as the group causing the only emergency withdrawal syndrome. Continuous use of drugs of this group produces a degree of dependence. Clearly the seriousness of that dependence relates not only to the dose, but also the duration of regular use and the consistency of that use. There is also a variation between different drugs with physical withdrawal symptoms being marked following continual consumption of barbiturates, alcohol and chlormethiazole. It is less prominent in the case of the benzodiazepines.

The Type Three user (as above) discontinuing a small, but long-term therapeutic dose of night sedation or a daytime tranquilliser is likely to experience symptoms of insomnia and moderate anxiety which are now understood to be withdrawal effects and not merely the recurrence of the original symptoms. The controlled user of a higher dose of benzodiazepines may experience more disturbing effects with restlessness and perceptual disturbance and sometimes depression. If the patient has been prescribed exceptionally high doses of a drug known to induce a significant physical dependence or has been obtaining additional supplies, it is preferable for withdrawal to be undertaken in hospital. Mild symptoms of insomnia, anxiety, restlessness and anorexia may progress to vomiting, hypotension, pyrexia, tremulousness, and in severe cases to major epileptic convulsions and/or organic confusional state with disorientation and hallucinations. This syndrome is, of course, well recognised as the delirium tremens usually associated with severe dependence on alcohol.

Management: The immediate management of severe withdrawals is to administer any convenient drug of this group. Diazepam orally, or in extreme cases, intramuscularly is most likely to be available in the general practitioner's emergency bag. The traditional longer-term in·patient management involved the administration of pentobarbital in divided doses to induce a mild degree of sedated intoxication, followed by a progressive withdrawal of approximately 100 mg daily. In the UK chlormethiazole has been advocated for withdrawal from drugs of this group, but it should only be used with extreme caution because of the likelihood of abuse. Supervision must be available to prevent the use of alcohol or other drugs, and its use limited to a period of not more than three weeks.

Where in-patient treatment is not available, or the patient has acceptable reasons to refuse admission, then the general practitioner may consider an attempt at out-patient withdrawal. The regime initiated in the Haigt Ashbury Clinic in San Francisco by Smith and Wesson has proved very satisfactory at the City Roads Crisis Intervention Unit, where there is nursing support available with only intermittent general practitioner attendance. Phenobarbitone should be administered in divided doses subject to a maximum of 300 mg in 24 hours, substituting 30 mg of phenobarbitone for 100 mg of medium-acting barbiturates. This dose is then reduced by incremental steps every second day over a period of 10 days to three weeks. Regular assessment is required and if the patient becomes agitated or tremulous then an increased dose will be required. If severe withdrawal symptoms appear transfer to hospital is recommended. Should epileptic convulsions occur then 10 mg of diazepam should be administered intramuscularly and an emergency ambulance summoned for immediate transfer to hospital. Where there has been multiple drug abuse, including benzodiazepines as well as other sedatives, then obviously a higher dose of phenobarbitone will be required than for withdrawal from barbiturates alone. Detailed advice is given in the appendices to the Guidelines of Good Clinical Practice in the Treatment of Drug Misuse published by the DHSS from which the Tables overleaf are reproduced[1]. It was sent to all medical practitioners and further copies may be available from District Health Authorities.

Withdrawal from benzodiazepines in therapeutic doses can be safely undertaken by a progressive reduction of the prescribed drug over a period of several weeks. Regular, brief surgery attendances will certainly be necessary for support. Some patients may require the additional support of a "tranquilliser support group" which may be available locally. In cases with severe anxiety referral direct to a psychologist may be appropriate.

Withdrawal from opiates

In a healthy person this situation is not physically life-threatening. The predominant and most pervasive symptom of opiate withdrawal is extreme anxiety and restlessness with a craving to obtain the drug, such that the patient may have recourse to undesirable activity such as purchasing illegal supplies. Other signs of opiate withdrawal are extremely variable and can generally be mimicked by an experienced drug user, they include runny nose and eyes, nausea, sometimes vomiting, diarrhoea and goose pimples. In carefully controlled studies of withdrawals these symptoms and signs do not always occur, but at the point where drugs are replaced by placebo, anxiety and sleep disturbance usually develop.

1.
The Editor and Author gratefully acknowledge permission given by the Controller of Her Majesty's Stationery Office to publish these tables.

Table 1 PHENOBARBITONE EQUIVALENTS FOR PRESCRIBING

Drug	Oral sedative dose	Equivalent phenobarbitone dose
Amylobarbitone (Amytal)	100 mg	30 mg
Butobarbitone (Soneryl)	100 mg	30 mg
Cyclobarbitone (Phanodorm)	200 mg	30 mg
Heptabarbitone (Medomin)	200 mg	30 mg
Quinalbarbitone (Seconal)	100 mg	30 mg
Quinalbarbitone and amylobarbitone (Tuinal)	50 mg + 50 mg	30 mg
Pentobarbitone (Nembutal)	100 mg	30 mg
Glutethimide (Doriden)	250 mg	30 mg
Methyprylone (Noludar)	200 mg	30 mg
Methaqualone* (illegally imported varieties)	250 mg	30mg

* No longer available in United Kingdom

Table 2 PHENOBARBITONE EQUIVALENT TO COMMON BENZODIAZEPINES

Benzodiazepines	Oral dose	Equivalent phenobarbitone dose
Chlordiazepoxide (Librium)	25 mg	30 mg
Clorazepate (Tranxene)	15 mg	30 mg
Diazepam (Valium)	15 mg	30 mg
Flurazepam (Dalmane)	30 mg	30 mg
Lorazepam (Ativan)	2 mg	30 mg
Oxazepam (Serenid)	10 mg	30 mg
Temazepam (Euhypnos, Normison)	30 mg	30 mg
Triazolam (Halcion)	0.125 mg	30 mg
Nitrazepam (Mogadon)	10 mg	30 mg
Medazepam (Nobrium)	10 mg	30 mg
Lormetazepam (Noctamid)	1 mg	30 mg
Laprazolam (Dormonoct)	2 mg	30 mg
Ketazolam (Anxon)	30 mg	30 mg
Flunitrazepam (Rohypnol)	1 mg	30 mg
Clobazam (Frisium)	10 mg	30 mg

Management of the patient in opiate withdrawal involves support and reassurance and occasionally prescription of a modest reducing dose of drugs. If a practitioner acquires the reputation for prescribing to temporary patients, then it has been the experience of those working in major conurbations that large numbers of patients may be attracted. It is suggested, therefore, that it is not appropriate to prescribe opioids to addicts in general practice except in three circumstances:

1. Where there is a serious concurrent medical or surgical condition and it is clearly inadvisable to superimpose the stress of withdrawal illness upon the physical condition.
2. Where a patient and their family are well known to a practitioner who has previously undertaken family medical care and is prepared, on a clear contractual basis, to assist an individual with the physical and psychological problems of withdrawal.
3. In exceptional circumstances where a patient has remained stable in receipt of maintenance prescription from a recognised treatment centre, then after full consultation it might be considered reasonable for a general practitioner to take over prescribing with continued support from the specialist centre.

Methadone mixture, drug tariff formula (see British National Formulary), is the drug of choice. Drugs should only be administered by injection in the very rare circumstances of a patient who is actually observed to be continuously vomiting. Tablets should never be prescribed for self-administration because of the probability of their being injected, with risk of local and sometimes systemic complications. Prescriptions **must** be organised so that dispensing is only on a basis of one or two days at a time; longer intervals between dispensing almost always results in over-use of drugs with recourse to alternative sources before the next prescription is due. Unless the patient is known to be a prolonged, heavy user of opioids, then a dose of 5-10 mg of methadone mixture, which may be repeated after two hours subject to a probable maximum of 20-25 mg, and an occasional maximum 24-hour consumption of 50 mg, is almost always sufficient to control withdrawal symptoms, although it may be less than the patient would wish to receive. It should always be made clear at the outset as to how long the practitioner is prepared to prescribe. For example, until an out-patient appointment can be obtained, or during the period when bed rest is required for the inter-current disorder. In the latter case it would generally be sensible and acceptable to offer a patient the opportunity then of a phased withdrawal over a period of two-three weeks subject to an understanding that they do not take other drugs. Minor tranquillisers should not be prescribed at the same time as methadone, except in the last few days and for a few weeks after a withdrawal course when careful administration of night sedation, but never on every night of the week, may be considered appropriate. A physician attending an opioid addict is required to notify the Chief Medical Officer at the Home Office (see British National

Formulary). A urine sample collected under observation from the patient, before commencement of any prescribing, provides some objective confirmation of the patient's account of what drugs they have been taking recently. In this context it should be noted that street drugs do not always contain the same substance as the consumer believes, and particularly when illegal supplies are difficult to obtain the patient may believe themselves to be addicted to opiates whereas in fact they have been consuming pharmaceutical tranquillisers presented as a powder.

For a more specific list of opioid equivalents for the purpose of prescribing to an addict refer to the Guidelines of Good Clinical Practice or to the booklet by Banks and Waller. (This is a practical guide and not a strict pharmacological analgesic equivalent.) Longer-term prescribing on a maintenance or extended withdrawal regime should not be undertaken in general practice, except after consultation with District or Regional specialist drug facilities who can provide back-up support, including laboratory testing facilities.

Withdrawal from stimulants

It should not be necessary to undertake any prescribing. Support and reassurance may be required. Sickness certification may be considered appropriate for persons who have been receiving long-term stimulants and are experiencing lethargy and hypersomnia, together with a degree of tension. Tricyclic antidepressants are not usually effective in combating any depression which occurs following withdrawal of stimulants. Monoamine oxidase inhibitors may be more effective, but there is a serious risk of hypertension, with a risk of cerebral haemorrhage if stimulants are consumed concurrently.

COMPLICATIONS OF DRUG MISUSE

The complications resulting from consumption of drugs other than alcohol, and possibly certain solvents, are primarily those associated with the mode of administration, the consequence of overdose, of accidents occurring while intoxicated, or the consumer neglecting their physical and social self-care. Of themselves the majority of the commonly misused drugs do not produce structural damage to the organs of the body through a direct toxic action. The Type Two drug user described above is at risk of placing the obtaining of drugs as a priority before many other social activities, including adequate nutrition or attention to hygiene and obtaining general medical care. Consumers of stimulants are often preoccupied with activities other than eating, a property utilised in the prescribing of these drugs to assist in weight reduction - a dubious practice not generally recommended!

Intravenous administration of drugs which contain adulterants and are not sterile can lead to septicaemia and endocarditis. The infection may sometimes be with exotic organisms and repeated bacteriological investigations may be required to isolate the infective agent. A series of cases of candidal endophthalmitis has been reported from Scotland and also noted on the continent of Europe, presumably due to contamination of self-injected heroin. The very property which renders the opioids so valuable in the management of terminal illness, and as an effective cough suppressant in appropriate chest conditions, can lead to the masking of symptoms of serious illness. The anxiety-relieving properties of the drug may lead the patient to ignore distressing symptoms which would normally lead to a medical consultation. The life-style of many addicts may also mean that they are not registered with a general practitioner and have considerable difficulty in persuading reception staff to arrange an urgent appointment. Every metropolitan casualty department can probably recall with embarrassment a small number of regular "nuisance" patients who at some point have complained of a pain in the chest or abdomen which the patients themselves, and staff, have attributed to withdrawal symptoms, but which have subsequently, and sadly on occasions only at post-mortems, been revealed to be due to such conditions as peritonitis from a ruptured appendix, pleurisy, staphylococcal pneumonia, etc. It is essential to undertake a physical examination, including recording of respiratory rate, pulse rate, temperature and blood pressure, in any addict complaining of any physical symptoms even when they themselves attribute these to withdrawals.

Syringe-transmitted infections

The majority of intravenous drug abusers presenting to Drug Clinics have evidence of serum (B) hepatitis and/or non-A, non-B hepatitis. A certain number of addicts are persistently Australia antigen positive indicating they are actively infectious; therefore, dressing of wounds, surgical and dental procedures must be undertaken with appropriate precautions. An assurance by the patient that they have never shared a syringe will usually be modified when it is pointed out that there is immunological evidence of previous infection. Hepatitis is usually acquired in the first year or two of intravenous drug use by the utilisation of a second-hand contaminated syringe or needle. There is little active treatment indicated, but bed rest is certainly advisable and since many addicts cannot have adequate care at home, referral to an infectious diseases unit is recommended.

The introduction of the HIV virus into the British addict population has now been clearly documented. This is particularly common in Scotland. Since the time course between infection with the virus and the development of serological markers is unknown, it is suggested that all body fluids from addicts should be treated as possibly infectious, at least until tested for virus antibody and with an assurance that the patient is not continuing to inject drugs. Advice regarding transmission of infection should be provided to families and residential facilities.

Local injection trauma

Long-term addicts who have sclerosed their accessible surface veins may inadvertently inject into arteries, particularly at elbow, wrist or in the groin. Injection of barbiturates in particular, is highly damaging to peripheral tissues and requires in-patient treatment. Perivenous, intramuscular and subcutaneous injections can give rise to local abscess formation. Caution should be exercised before incising fluctuant swellings, particularly in the groin, because of the occasional development of a traumatic arterial aneurysm following self-injection.

PREGNANCY AND DRUG ADDICTION

Evidence regarding the risk to the fetus where the mother consumes drugs during pregnancy is somewhat confused. There is no doubt that there is an increased perinatal mortality amongst babies born to obvious Type Two drug users. Certainly many psychoactive drugs cross the placenta and the baby may be born with a degree of physical dependence which will require treatment. It is, however, probable that many of the complications occurring in the neonatal period are related to the poor nutrition and inadequate prenatal care of the mother during the pregnancy.

Management: Ensure that hospital based prenatal care is attended by patient and inform hospital of patient's drug use. The widespread belief amongst addicts that if they admit to their problem, then Social Services may intervene to take the newborn child into care, is a reason why pregnant mothers conceal their drug use. In most areas Social Services attempt to support addicted parents with a young child. Certainly many addicts prove to be adequate parents. On occasions, however, the child may need to be placed on the At Risk Register and a case conference held. If Care proceedings are considered for the protection of the child, these should be based on objective evidence that the parent's behaviour is a risk to the child.

COUNSELLING REGARDING DRUG PROBLEMS

This should not be undertaken as an emergency although panic stricken relatives are likely to regard such a matter as of extreme urgency. Unless there is an overdose situation, the patient is suffering from panic reactions, or is in severe withdrawal, then it is preferable to set time aside for a proper consideration of the psychological and social situation, as well as time to take a detailed drug history. In a handbook on emergency treatment this topic cannot be considered adequately. There are now an increasing number of organisations able to provide some immediate telephone advice, and usually to arrange a personal meeting for counselling. Such organisations are either staffed by volunteers or salaried staff who are not medical practitioners. Many such organisations, however, have access to and support from specialised NHS drug facilities. Unless a general practitioner feels confident regarding the misuse of illegal drugs, it is probable that the experience and training of persons in these services renders them the most appropriate agency for counselling; on the other hand the status and confidence inspired by an established family practitioner is of great importance in any such counselling situation. Many such organisations now offer brief courses which can familiarise medical practitioners with the likely drugs that are being abused in a locality and with local information regarding alternative treatment facilities and are reasonably adept at developing a collaborative counselling programme with the family doctor.

Where drug use is only intermittent and conforms to Type One, as described above, then information regarding the **possible** hazards associated with drug use, and the handing over of an information sheet such as the pamphlet Drug Misuse, A Basic Briefing produced by the DHSS as a guide to professionals, parents and others who need to know more about drugs and their effects, may be sufficient. Supplies will be available for distribution in GP surgeries through District Health Authorities most probably the Health Education Service. In offering advice, in addition to ascertaining what drugs and with what frequency they are consumed, it is extremely important to understand what function drug taking may perform in relation to other members of the family or referring organisation. In the institutional setting it may be appropriate to understand drug misuse as behaviour comparable to self-injury, or setting fires, rather than as a pharmacological problem. As in any counselling situation it is important to avoid being censorious or adopting too directive a technique. This need not prevent the practitioner maintaining a clear personal standpoint regarding drug taking as a potentially hazardous procedure; such a view-point will be more convincing if alcohol and nicotine are clearly referred to as drugs of addiction.

REFERENCES

1. Banks, A. and Waller, T.A.N. (1983). Drug Addiction and Polydrug Abuse: The Role of the General Practitioner. Institute for the Study of Drug Dependence: London
2. Mitcheson, M. (1983). Drug addiction. In Oxford Textbook of Medicine. Oxford University Press: Oxford
3. Thorley, A. (19??). Managing the opiate drug taker: The general practitioner's role. Medicine in Practice, 26, 666-673 (SCODA)

Facts about AIDS for drug users; HELPLINE 01-833 2971: The Standing Conference on Drug Abuse with The Terrence Higgins Trust: DHSS. Drug Misuse - A Basic Briefing: DM3 DHSS 1985

19

Excited patients

John B Loudon

QUICK REFERENCE GUIDE

THE SORTING PROCESS

Scheme of approach:
Is the excitement new or is it recurrent?

A. New excitement

   i. Is it a response to a recent life event?
   ii. Has it occurred against a background of strange or altered behaviour?
   iii. Is there any evidence of experimentation with drugs?
   iv. Has a new treatment just been prescribed?
   v. Have drugs recently been withdrawn?

B. Recurrent excitement

   i. Is there a history of repeated inappropriate responses to times of crisis in the patient's life?
   ii. Is there a history of repeated psychiatric admissions?
   iii. Is there a history of long-standing abuse of drugs?

C. **Assessment**

D. **Management**   Psychological
                     Pharmacological

E. **Forensic considerations**

Excitement can be psychological or neurophysiological in origin, and can be induced pharmacologically. Psychologically, the term refers to arousal of perceptions and drives, with the expectation of gratification of these strong needs. The thought of the object or wish which is arousing excitement predominates in the mind, obliterating all other considerations. Physiologically, the term emphasises arousal of nervous mechanisms so that even small stimuli may produce strong responses. There is no habituation to novel events and reactions may be quite out of keeping. In such a state of arousal, the individual's conscious experience will be coloured by his state of mind so that frustration or anger may give rise to strong paranoid feelings or a sense of loss or failure to depressive ideation.

Drugs which suppress self control, or which excite arousal may produce excited states which will last in accordance with the duration of action of the drug in the body. The excited patient is someone whose ability to perceive reality is temporarily impaired. Excitement has aroused in him a strength of feeling or expectation which is out of keeping with actuality. The onlooker may be implicated. This may be as an object of the desire or as a person who is frustrating a course of action which is self evidently right for the patient. As a result of the strength of excitement normal caution and inhibitions may fail to control behaviour. It is difficult to think of a state of excitement being normal for the individual.

A. **EXCITEMENT NEW FOR THAT PARTICULAR PATIENT**

i. **Life events**

As a result of early experiences all of us have memories of particular people or events which meant a lot to us and who in memory were the cause of satisfying experiences for us. There are some for whom that supply of good experiences was insufficient or was cut off prematurely, leaving a sense of longing which has persisted in the background, often unacknowledged. As time goes by the longing will become increasingly inappropriate. At times of particular crisis, there is an inevitable arousal of feelings and coping strategies are tested. If the individual is unable to cope with what is threatened, he may revert to a frame of mind appropriate to an earlier time. The unassuaged longing may come forth. A person in the present may be cast as the object of this longing, and the feeling is often strongly sexualised.

ii. Against a background of altered behaviour

As a serious mental disorder is brewing, there are often no major external signs that something is amiss. The individual may seem a little withdrawn or strange, and may feel this himself. However, habit and routine will often serve to keep his behaviour superficially normal. The incurious among family, friends or colleagues detect no change. A sudden florid burst of symptoms, alarming to those around the patient may still not be seen in retrospect to have been preceeded by a change. Careful inquiry may reveal evidence of change. Such excitement may include exalted or dysphoric mood, psychotic symptoms such as delusion formation and over-activity, and may be part of a schizophrenic or manic condition. A patient suffering from morbid jealousy may also suddenly launch into activity having been brooding awhile on the imagined wrongs of the spouse. Similarly, a patient suffering from a demented condition, aware of failing powers and reacting to imperfect memory by suspicion, may respond with gross arousal to any change in circumstances. This may be a change of house or an illness of the main care giver.

iii. Is there evidence of experimentation with drugs?

Many drugs of abuse can produce excited states. Solvent inhalation or the sniffing of gas lighter refills produces an acute intoxication, during which violent acts or serious self-injurious behaviour may occur. This seems to be as a result of alteration of brain structure produced by the lipid solvent nature of some of the compounds used, or by anoxia. Nervous systems depending on the chemical dopamine seem to have functions which correspond to behaviour showing drive or goal-directed actions. In their extreme form this would be called excitement. Cocaine and amphetamines both release dopamine which stimulates these systems and frequently produces excited states, often followed by compensatory lethargy. Other drugs may engender false experiences and the individual may become aroused and overactive. Heavy cannabis use and exposure to LSD both may alter and falsify experience to such an extent that excitement results.

iv. New treatment

If an individual, never known before to have become disturbed or excited, develops such behaviour just after starting a new treatment then the treatment must be implicated as a cause of the disturbance. The effect may be as a result of therapeutic action, as from tricyclic antidepressant or from a strongly stimulating monoamine oxidase inhibitor such as tranylcypromine. Otherwise it could be a known side effect, such as akathisia or the patient's reaction to an acute dystonia, both from neuroleptic drugs. Finally, it might be due to a delirium as a result of toxicity or an interaction between two drugs, such as the atropinic type of poisoning resulting from an interaction between antiparkinsonian drugs and chlorpromazine.

v. Drug withdrawal

Certain drugs suppress cerebral functions; the barbiturates benzodiazepines, alcohol and opiates are prominent in this respect. Abrupt withdrawal of such drugs will be followed by a resurgence of the cerebral function suppressed. The strength of this will be determined by the extent to which it was originally suppressed, and by the rapidity with which the drug is cleared from the brain. Alcohol, and short acting barbiturates and benzodiazepines leave the brain in a few hours; longer acting drugs such as diazepam may result in an attenuated reaction several days later as they are withdrawn. Again, the individual's frame of mind and the severity of the reaction will determine what emotional colouration is experienced and the extent to which excitement develops.

B. RECURRENT EPISODES OF EXCITEMENT

i. Is there a pattern at times of crisis?

Some individuals, apparently of even temperament in normal times, show a bewildering change at times of difficulty or crisis. It is then that ways of coping are put to the test and their value becomes apparent. At such a time we all feel a sense of arousal which may be manifested by interrupted sleep or some difficulty in concentrating. For some, the potential change may so disorganise the individual that his arousal becomes even greater and an excited state supervenes. Those who know him well will recollect previous episodes and should be able to relate it to circumstances. From time to time any practitioner will come across individuals who seem to generate excitement around them. These will often be personally disordered people. They exist emotionally by vicariously stimulating responses and feelings in those around them. These are often the vulnerable and weak, who may be driven to a frenzy of feeling entirely beyond their ability to cope.

ii. Is there a history of repeated psychiatric illnesses?

Excitement can form part of the symptom picture of a recurrent manic or schizophrenic illness and may well be the sole presenting symptom. However, a history of previous contact with psychiatrists, a reaction on the part of the patient to the suggestion of a psychiatric referral or the finding of prescribed psychotropic drugs must give rise to the suspicion of a recurring psychiatric illness.

iii. Excitement in long-standing abusers of drugs

Although habitual users of drugs may be expected to be used to their favourite compound, vagaries of supply and an absence of quality control mean that regularity of use and potency cannot be assumed. Also a tendency to experiment, to try new compounds, or new combinations, are all part of the drug user's repertoire. It would be safe to assume that excitement occurring in this population will be of drug origin until proved otherwise. Urine screening allows a means of finding out which compound or compounds are implicated.

C. Assessment

Given the furore which the excited patient may cause before a doctor is called, accurate assessment may be very difficult. Those near to the patient may be very upset, pushed into responses which make the situation worse, and may have involved the police which will have its own effect. The prevailing feeling will depend on whether the excited patient is being viewed as "mad" or "bad". This will also determine how tolerant people will be. Either way the patient is likely to be alienated from those around, beyond his own control but perhaps frightened by the events he has set in train. For the attending doctor to be effective in bridging this gap it is important that his contact with the patient is qualitatively different from angry relatives or minatory police. This means avoiding threats, being willing to listen, perhaps at some length, and remaining calm. However, there is no obligation to put personal safety at risk.

To a large extent, the outcome will depend on the command of the situation the doctor can impose as a result of the expectations others will have of him. Imposing his order will allow assessment properly to take place. In addition to some account from the patient, a history will be needed from a friend or relative. Details of compounds ingested, whether licit or illicit will be very important. Past medical and psychiatric history will give important clues. News of life events or recent experiences will be important to give an insight into how the patient may be feeling. This will also give an opening for rapport to be established with the patient. Any physical examination possible will concentrate on signs or symptoms of intoxication.

Three factors - evidence of a psychiatric syndrome, suggestions as to how orientated the patient is, and how amenable he is to discussion - will hint at avenues of treatment.

D. **Treatment**

i. **Psychological**

An attempt at psychological management will succeed or fail depending on to what extent the patient can be reached by normal human communication. Someone who acknowledges the doctor's presence, who realises his profession, who maintains some eye contact, who can engage in discussion, and who can accept assurances of care is likely to respond to sincerity, warmth and a willingness to listen. An ability to think oneself into the patient's shoes, to try to empathise with what is known about the patient's predicament will engender trust. Deft use of what is known about the patient's family circle and friends, his interests and goals will often reinforce normal controls of his behaviour. The doctor must be prepared to be tested out by the patient who may try a little threatening behaviour to see how easily he can be thrown, or intimidated as others may have been. The aim must be to present oneself as a path to a relationship with the world. This should promise to be more rewarding in the long term than the short term gains of the excited but alienated position the patient has got himself into. Therefore threats and warnings about consequences are of little use. Such negative reinforcers are generally poor at modifying behaviour. Much more effective are promises of rewards and hints of the doctor's own warm regard if the patient accepts his invitation to talk and not act on the problems which are bothering him.

ii. **Physical methods**

On the premise that underlying excitement is an overarousal of the nervous system, drug treatment can be used to dampen down arousal thus reducing the excitement.

a. **Benzodiazepines**: Such drugs, given by mouth or parenterally, have the major advantages that they are particularly non-toxic especially in the short term. Apart from sedation there are very few side-effects. As they act only on a particular receptor site in the brain, and have no non-specific effect, there is unlikely to be any accumulation of action in synergy with other cerebral depressants the patient has taken.

For rapid oral action, diazepam 10-20 mg, lorazepam 2.5-5 mg or temazepam 40-60 mg are to be preferred. (Chlordiazepoxide and oxazepam are absorbed more slowly.) The dose can be repeated in 30-45 minutes if no effect is observed.

If the parenteral route is preferred, lorazepam 3-6 mg or a special preparation of diazepam (Diazemuls) 10-20 mg are suitable, and may be repeated after 15-30 minutes.

(Standard parenteral preparations of diazepam are poorly absorbed from intramuscular injection.)

b. **Neuroleptics**: use of these drugs carries the risk of precipitating dystonia and severe extrapyramidal side effects, which in themselves are dangerous, and may fuel the patient's excitement. Chlorpromazine may produce profound hypotension which can be a source of injury to the patient, and its effect, even from a single dose, may persist for over 24 hours.

Droperidol is a potent sedative neuroleptic with the **advantage of a short duration of action** which allows better titration of the dose to the patient's condition. In the short term **it rarely causes extrapyramidal side effects, and cardiovascular problems are rare**. Dosage at 10-20 mg orally and 5-10 mg parenterally can be repeated every 30 minutes until control is achieved. If neuroleptics are used, parenteral anti-Parkinsonian drugs, such as orphenadrine or procyclidine, should be available.

Paraldehyde is now an archaic treatment for excitement or disturbed behaviour, although it had the merit of great safety. The pain of the injection, the fumes the patient breathed out for the next day or two, and the need for glass syringes excludes it from modern practice.

In treating excitement with drugs, there is nothing to be gained by switching from one compound to another. All patients will respond at some point to any of the drugs described above. The trick is to carry on with one compound while observing for signs of impending toxicity.

E. FORENSIC CONSIDERATIONS

Giving medication parenterally to an excited patient means some degree of compulsion. **Resort to the Mental Health Act is not necessary if it can be shown that the doctor's obligations under common law required the use of medication to prevent serious harm to the patient or others**. Giving parenteral medication to an excited patient on one's own is not to be recommended. At the same time it may not be necessary to overwhelm the patient with numbers of bodies. Sufficient force in the background, a clearly expressed determination to get medication into the patient by mouth, or failing that, by injection, may be enough to realise some co-operation from the patient, despite his disturbed mental state.

20

Confused patients

Michael Swash

QUICK REFERENCE GUIDE

The term **confusion** is often used, not only in a medical sense, but as an everyday term in ordinary conversation. As such it is not strictly defined. This is unfortunate, for the development of a confusional state in the medical sense, referred to as **delirium**, always means that the specific and unmistakeable psychological symptoms produced are due to an organic lesion, metabolic or chemical effect on the brain. The term confusion is also used in a loose sense to denote **dementia which is best defined as a syndrome of global disturbance of higher mental function occurring in an alert patient.** It is important to recognise that dementia may be static or progressive, reversible or irreversible; these aspects depend on its cause, treatment, or any association with other extraneous factors (see also p.15).

   Delirium, a syndrome of global disturbance of mental function occurring in association with clouding of consciousness, is not uncommon in patients with dementia but also occurs as an acute disorder, formerly termed acute confusional state. Delirium occurs as an acute or subacute illness characterised by hallucinations, especially visual hallucinations, and restlessness. It often develops in the context of a sudden change in environment, as during hospitalisation for investigation, or during an intercurrent illness. Delirium thus quite frequently complicates dementia and may, indeed, be the presenting feature of an otherwise inapparent dementia.

The psychological symptoms of delirium can be the first evidence of a brain lesion (e.g. acute meningitis) and, as the vast majority of the conditions causing it are remediable, a full search for these should be made. Early treatment is necessary to avoid permanent brain impairment and the supervention of dementia. It is easy to fail to distinguish this important development from uncomplicated dementia or a functional disturbance, so that its urgency remains undetected.

The symptoms of delirium are stereotyped, but the rate of onset is important, for whereas hypothyroidism or Cushing's syndrome can cause subacute or chronic confusional states, high fever from whatever cause will produce an acute, urgent condition.

SYMPTOMS AND SIGNS OF DELIRIUM

1. **Clouding of consciousness.** The patient is neither somnolent nor fully alert. The level of awareness fluctuates, causing different appearances in the patient's behaviour, in short periods of time. There are sudden changes in mental function, often taking the form of noisy, inconsequential behavioural responses. Between episodes of noisy lack of self-control the patient becomes drowsy or shows clouding of consciousness again. A patient said to have been totally disorientated half an hour previously may seem completely rational during a brief interview later, only to relapse shortly afterwards. It is important not to miss this variation as it always means an organic problem and the exclusion of functional psychoses such as schizophrenia, in which consciousness remains clear and unvarying.

2. **Disorientation** for time, person and place is usually shown. The patient does not recognise his environment and may misidentify relatives and friends. Diminution of level of awareness leads to loss of the sense of passage of time.

3. **Memory disturbance** is inevitable. It covers the period of confusion during which perception and registration are grossly impaired.

4. **Perception is impaired** and distorted and, whereas visual hallucinations are uncommon in functional psychoses, they are common in confusional states. Illusions are common: a feeling of dizziness is felt as "someone rocking the bed"; the telephone ringing is heard as an alarm of some kind; the wallpaper design is seen as "coloured elephants".

5. **Fragmentation of speech and thought** is characteristic. Words are properly spoken but disconnected to form a meaningless utterance. The patient cannot express thoughts properly nor cooperate.

6. **Mood variation**. The characteristic mood in delirium is fear, but it can range from restless excitability to jocularity (see also p.83).

ACUTE DEVELOPMENTS IN CHRONIC CONFUSED PATIENTS

Here, emphasis is given to the common acute conditions, but in relation to investigation it is worth remembering that acute confusion can arise often in the setting of a subacute or chronic state (e.g. influenza in the setting of myxoedema, or haemorrhage into a slowly growing cerebral tumour).

CAUSES OF CONFUSIONAL STATES

A. **Effects of drugs** (see pages 188-203)

Alcohol
Benzodiazepines
Barbiturates
Bromides
Tricyclic antidepressants (especially in the elderly)
Digitalis
Anti-Parkinsonian agents
LSD and other hallucinogens
"Glue" and various inhalants
Opiates

B. **Infections**

a. Systemic infections producing toxic effects and high pyrexia
   e.g. pneumonia, typhoid, malaria, septicaemia
b. Brain and meninges
   e.g. meningitis, encephalitis, cerebral abscess

C. **Sudden withdrawal of drugs**

e.g. withdrawal of alcohol, benzodiazepines, barbiturates

D. **Metabolic disturbance**

e.g.   Hypoglycaemia, hyperglycaemia
Hypothyroidism
Anoxia
Uraemia
Hepatic failure
Deficiency of vitamins B_1, B_6 or B_{12}
Cushing's syndrome
Hypopituitarism
Use of corticosteroids
Hypocalcaemia

E. **Organic brain damage**

a. Head injury. Concussion
b. Vascular accidents.   Cerebral thrombus and embolism
Haemorrhage into neoplasm
Subarachnoid haemorrhage
Subdural haematoma
c. Intracranial neoplasm, primary or secondary
d. Raised intracranial pressure from any cause.

F. **Factors causing delirium in the setting of pre-existing dementia**

a. Pain
    i. Abdominal
    ii. Renal
    iii. Limb (fractures)
b. Sensory deprivation
    i. Blindness
    ii. Deafness
    iii. Language problem
c. Perceptual isolation
    i. Hospitalisation
    ii. Anaesthesia
    iii. Bereavement
    iv. Environmental change
d. Alcohol intoxication
e. Depressive illness with retardation.

DELIRIUM IN CHILDREN AND ADULTS

Delirium occurs in children and healthy young adults in the face of overwhelming systemic disease, such as pneumonia or acute severe metabolic processes, for example hypercalcaemia, uraemia, or drug intoxications. In these instances delirium does not necessarily imply the presence of any fixed structural or biochemical brain disorder, and the condition is reversible by appropriate treatment of the underlying cause.

214

DELIRIUM IN THE ELDERLY

In the elderly, delirium is a common presentation of systemic disease. Pneumonia, meningitis, urinary tract infection, diarrhoea, or metabolic disorders are common causes. Also, presentation with delirium usually indicates not only an acute disturbance requiring treatment, but the presence of mild underlying dementia. Delirious states thus usually represent the superimposition of another illness on an underlying disorder of mental function, although sometimes they may occur as a consequence of a rapid deterioration in an underlying disease process. For example, in multifocal vascular disease delirium may occur with the advent of further infarction. Delirium also occurs commonly as a manifestation of occult minor seizures, for example in patients with tumours and, less commonly, in patients with underlying epilepsy that is poorly controlled.

Delirium may also develop in response to severe or continued pain in elderly people and treatment of the underlying pain, for example from an occult fracture, may result in marked improvement in the mental state.

The **perceptual isolation** of hospitalisation, or of bereavement, is a common cause of rapid decline in mental function in the elderly. This must be recognised by the appearance of bizarre behavioural symptoms and treated by restoration of social contact, and not by sedation with tranquilliser or neuroleptic medications. The latter are likely to produce long-term side-effects and may, even in the short term, result in deterioration in mental function rather than improvement.

Drugs, and alcoholism are major demographic causes of impaired mental function in the elderly. This cause may not be recognised if the history of hypnotic, tranquilliser or neuroleptic therapy is not available to the clinician. The patient may be using these drugs as a means of obtaining relief from intolerable symptoms, for example depression or insomnia, or by sharing the medication with another patient for whom a prescription has been given entirely appropriately.

The appearance of an acute confusional state in an elderly subject carries the need for investigation to establish cause, and then effective treatment. When the patient has recovered, the possibility of an underlying defect of intellectual processing, due to early dementia, must be considered.

If dementia is present, further investigation is necessary to exclude metabolic causes such as hypothyroidism, hypovitaminosis, cerebral tumour, or hydrocephalus. Alzheimer's senile dementia remains, at present, a diagnosis made on a combination of positive features in the history and examination, and negative features, implying the absence of any other treatable or untreatable cause of global impairment of mental function (see pp.165,166).

MENTAL STATUS TESTING

A large number of different systems for mental status testing have been suggested for clinical use. Most of these tests are loosely derived from standard tests used by psychologists in clinical practice and, as such, they may be taken only as a loose guide to mental function since they are taken out of context from the numerical background of the psychological test procedure.

One commonly used test is the mental status questionnaire. This test consists of **ten simple questions** indicating alertness, orientation for time and place, and recent and remote memory. These ten questions need not be asked of the patient in serial order but can be placed naturally in the process of examination (Table 1). All normal subjects should score correct answers in nine or ten of the questions and scores of less than eight imply some degree of confusion.

Table 1 MENTAL STATUS QUESTIONNAIRE

---

1. What is the name of this place (where are we now)?
2. What is the address of this place?
3. What is the date?
4. What month is it?
5. What year is it?
6. How old are you?
7. When is your birthday?
8. What year were you born?
9. Who is the Prime Minister?
10. Who was the previous Prime Minister?

More complex questions, derived from the Wechsler adult intelligence scale (WAIS), involve testing a patient's memory for an address after a minute or more of abstraction, testing memory for a list of unrelated items immediately and after abstraction, serially subtracting 7 from 100 (a test that implies normal recent memory as well as calculational abilities), proverb interpretation, and descriptions of the information content of simple cartoon-like drawings. Tests of this nature require some experience for their appropriate interpretation. It is wise for the clinician to **develop a few tests on these lines** and to use them constantly from patient to patient in order to allow assessment of their value.

Questions concerning the patient's ability to care for himself at home, in terms of cooking, dressing, shopping, going out alone, and bathing, and in relation to continence, are important general questions providing a clear idea of the patient's mobility and intellectual functioning.

Finally, **the face/hand test has been much used in the assessment of** patients with dementia and delirium. In this test the patient is asked to sit with his eyes closed and his hands on his knees. The examiner strokes the patient's cheek and, at the same time, one hand. Alternate combinations of face and hand may be touched and on each occasion the patient is asked to report the contact. Incorrect answers are associated with organic disease; the patient with functional disorders performs normally in this test.

DIFFERENTIAL DIAGNOSIS

Delirium should be distinguished from:
1. The "confusion" produced by **psychological overload**.
2. The "confusion" caused by confusing circumstances in the environment.
3. The psychological picture of uncomplicated dementia.
4. Functional and drug-induced psychoses, particularly depressive illness.

1. **Emotional overload**: The individual is so tense, overwrought or fussed already that new additional exciting or emotional developments cause **a sense of disturbance of thinking**. The individual has full insight into this and it causes him or her additional anguish. Very often the experience is expressed as "I couldn't think straight", "I was absolutely dumbfounded", "My mind boggled". Most students have had similar experiences in very tense situations such as viva voce examinations. A harmless question is asked and although the candidate knows the answer, he or she cannot think of the appropriate reply, terms or phrases at the time. The answer, comes shortly after leaving the examination hall, when relaxing with other "sufferers".

   The characteristics of this state are that it is usually **short-lived**, related to **specific stress** and, into which **the person has insight**. However, in very vulnerable individuals of marked sensitivity, continual emotional overload can lead to hysterical symptoms in which an element of subjective confusion is prominent (see also p.58).

2. **Confusing circumstances**: The patient feels a sense of "confusion" because in the absence of a formal psychological illness he cannot make out clearly in a psychological sense what is going on around him. Those associating with the patient make vague statements which convey no indication of intention, feeling or conviction. A feeling of mistrust develops in which even obvious factual statements are disbelieved. Exemplified in Kafka's **The Trial**, the individual, deprived of facilities for testing the reality of what he hears, becomes uncertain, lacking in confidence and "confused". It is **characterised by full insight**, the absence of **psychiatric disorder** such as paranoid psychosis and the existence of **uncertainty** or the expression of uncertainty in the human environment.

3. **Dementia**: Delirium should be distinguished from uncomplicated dementia. Clouding of consciousness and fluctuation in the level of awareness are two features of delirium which can be quickly recognised and which separate it from uncomplicated dementia. In the elderly, as mentioned earlier, delirium is usually super-imposed on an underlying dementia.

4. **Functional and drug-induced psychoses**: Non-organic disorders of mental function, particularly the development of psychotic illness, especially **depression or drug-induced psychosis,** such as that due to steroid therapy, must not be neglected. Especially in the elderly, **depression is a common and serious cause of debility and illness**. The depressed patient is difficult to assess and may not respond in a full and compliant manner to mental status testing so that full investigation and examination is difficult. Reliance on incomplete data in the establishment of a diagnosis is unwise in any branch of medicine and this is particularly so in the investigation of a confused patient. If there is difficulty in assessing the patient the examiner should ask himself whether this reflects not so much his own inadequacies in establishing contact with the patient, as a disorder in the patient's mood. Serious depressive illness may escape notice if the clinician becomes over concerned with details of the process of development of an illness and if a moment is not spared for an overall assessment of the patient's bearing, dress, attitude and social contacts.

INVESTIGATIONS

Investigations designed to consider possible diagnoses listed earlier may be applied to patients with confusion, but these tests should be used economically and appropriately. **Clinical assessment, and examination, will often give a clue to the underlying cause and** it should thus be possible to decide on a rational series of investigations, without screening every patient for every conceivable cause of impaired mental functioning. Economy of investigation is an aim that is appropriate not only for the economics of health care, but for the patient. It should not be necessary to raise anxiety levels, or involve the patient in a large number of complex and expensive investigations involving many visits to hospital departments for strange tests and manipulations before deciding on an appropriate means of treatment.

MANAGEMENT

Appropriate management is dependent upon appropriate assessment. In many patients contact with other people and placement in an appropriate context and environment will be sufficient to improve mental state. In others, judicious use of neuroleptic medication, for example thioridazine, chlorpromazine or diazepam will be useful. Treatment of an underlying cause, particularly in patients with delirium, is an essential aim, sometimes unrealised in practice because of the multifactorial nature of the underlying functional disturbance. In younger people assiduous search for metabolic disorders, or for drug effects, is often rewarding. In the elderly, occult infections, painful disorders, bereavement unknown to the doctor, or perceptual isolation are common.

21

Moody patients

John D Pollitt

THE SORTING PROCESS

Is the moodiness lifelong or recent?

A. **Lifelong moodiness**

    i. Is it diurnal? Consider: Normal diurnal moodiness or if exaggerated, **depressive illness.**

    ii. Is the individual emotionally immature? Consider: **Hysterical, sensitive personality**.

iii. Is the individual unreliable, unstable, unpredictable and unable to take responsibility? Consider: **Psychopathic personality**.

iv. Does the individual show relatively long periods of either gloominess and sadness or high spirits and elation? Consider: **Cyclothymic personality**.

B. **Recent moodiness**

i. Is there a recent disturbance of sleep, appetite, weight, libido and outlook on self and/or the world? Consider: **Depressive illness**.

ii. Has there been a recent change towards high spirits, overactivity, tirelessness and talkativeness? Consider: **Hypomania**.

iii. Is there a divergence between topic and the emotion expressed (incongruity of affect) coupled with social withdrawal, bizarre delusions, auditory hallucinations and feelings of being influenced or supernaturally affected? Consider: **Schizophrenia**.

iv. Have intracranial lesions and cerebral infections of all kinds been carefully considered and (where appropriate) investigated? Consider: **Slow growing cerebral tumours** (meningiomas), **secondary metastatic deposits, intracranial infections**.

v. Could an endocrine disorder be responsible? If so is it acute or chronic?

a. Acute mood changes - Consider: **Premenstrual syndrome** or **hypoglycaemia**.

b. Chronic mood changes - Consider: **Myxoedema, hyperthyroidism, Cushing's syndrome, Addison's disease** or **parathyroid disease**.

vi. Has a hormone been administererd? Consider: **Oral contraceptive** or **corticosteroids**.

vii. Are drugs responsible? If so are they self chosen or prescribed?
Self-chosen - Consider: **LSD, cocaine, solvents, amphetamines**.
Prescribed - Consider: **Imipramine, tranylcypromine**.

viii. Has a marked change in biological rhythm been imposed recently? Consider: **Unsatisfactory shift work, moonlighting, imposed sleep disturbance, flying through time zones, excessive persistent dieting**.

Moodiness is common in the population but because there is considerable tolerance of moodiness and people rarely have insight into this trait it is not a common presenting problem.

It can, however, assume psychotic proportions and demand immediate intervention. In many cases emergency situations stem from mood changes.

It may point to a reversible disturbance which if untreated may cause the break-up of the family or friendships while communications of all types suffer.

It should be a subject of further investigations whenever the suspicion arises.

Even when moodiness is recognised it is often attributed to current circumstances and the result of the mood can often be mistaken for the cause. The patient rationalises his or her behaviour in terms of current problem and the possibility of other factors is overlooked.

The key question is **"Has the individual changed?"** The first stage in sorting out the nature of moodiness is to separate the patient who is and has always been moody from the person who has recently become moody. This separation is important because without exception something can be done for all those in the latter group.

A. MOODINESS AS A LIFELONG PERSONAL ATTRIBUTE

i. Diurnal variation

The first variety of mood change is found in almost everyone. It is the diurnal variation in mood of healthy people, usually manifest either as tiredness, slowness, lethargy or even low-spirits in the morning to be followed by a steady shift in mood after mid-morning, which leads to a sense of cheerfulness in the evening. We are often unaware of the difference in ourselves, but the well accepted wisdom of popping the question in the evening or discussing a sensitive issue over an evening meal indicates the commoner trend of feeling heartiest in the latter half of the day.

These changes have to be distinguished from the diurnal swing of mood seen in depressive illness. In the latter there is invariably a sleep disturbance, which is not present in otherwise healthy people.

ii. The hysterical personality (see also Chapter 7)

An unfortunate name with many meanings is the only accepted label for a group of traits met n both sexes quite commonly in the general healthy population. An unexpected turn of events upsets such people unduly, for they are easily hurt or disappointed and tend to show clearly that they have been "put out". Such mood changes are rapid, often starting suddenly and dramatically when something goes wrong. An innocent comment is "taken the wrong way" or it is felt that the latest request is "the last straw" and quite unreasonable.

Such people are thought to have delayed emotional development and are still, whatever the chronological age, arrested during adolescence. Some are shy, withdrawn as young prepubertal children, while others are tough, dominating and bossy individuals, more reminiscent of the 5th or lower 6th form at school, but all are sensitive, emotional and sometimes superficial, tending to dramatise

222

their assets and moans and finding difficulty in peer relationships. This difficulty arises from a tendency either to dominate and control or to take an opposite stance of "Poor little me". Both attitudes tend to manipulate others, forcing them to comply in an emotional way rather than a rational one.

Friendships tend to be fickle and there is above average gullibility and suggestibility. Artistic qualities are well represented and there is often an artistic flair which singles out the patient in a group.

In ordinary conversation there is often a naturalness and forthcoming, open attitude which can be complicated by an unintended seductive quality. Stories are heightened by the use of superlatives, everything is marvellous and newly met acquaintances are welcomed by first names, or overfamiliarly as "darling". In argument there is an all or nothing quality about the person's attitudes.

In personal appearance the markedly hysterical personality stands out in two ways. Firstly, their sense of dress and drama enhances their appearance in a pleasing artistic (or perhaps shocking) way and, secondly, their youthful looks last even into middle life, the fineness of skin texture and their general physical agelessness allow them an advantage envied particularly by older women. This, in association with tendencies to dramatise, with good verbal communication, and sometimes ready familiarity, early in the professional relationship, assist the detection of this personality in the consulting room.

iii. Sociopathic or psychopathic personality

In some psychopaths, there is poor mood control and **they react quickly** to immediate circumstances. This changeability of mood leads to the label of "unstable psychopath". In such people mood variation can be extreme and fluctuate wildly. Control is further impaired by alcohol, so that a few drinks can lead them to become noisy, quarrelsome, violent and even savagely destructive.

The problem is one of failure of development or extremely slow development, so that those affected do not develop a social conscience or those sentiments which govern conduct. They tend to be impulsive. Consequently, although a proportion show slow improvement, this might be expected by the age of 40 or 50. Until that time their dominant character traits are antisocial showing either an inadequate, aggressive or pseudo-artistic quality overall.

Detection of this personality type depends on the history rather than the individual's story. A history of drifting, lack of ambition, emotional instability and violence is highly suggestive. Other features include a failure to learn, lack of values, selfishness, and an inability to forego present pleasure for future gain.

They can be affectionless, egocentric and demanding, and they show little guilt, anxiety or remorse. They do not form stable emotional relationships and show no realistic ambition or foresight.

Often restless, they do not profit from experience or punishment and are frequently impulsive, lacking the awareness of others' needs.

In the surgery appearances in this group can be highly deceptive for they are plausible, likeable and natural. Without a proper history the doctor can easily be misled by distortions which occasionally amount to pathological lying, so that the first realisation of the true nature of the problem is the evidence of unreliability in the patient's behaviour.

iv. Cyclothymic personality

The mood changes found in cyclothymic personalities differ from those seen in hysterical and sociopathic personalities in that the **mood deviation lasts much longer.**

Whereas a hysterical person may show tears, resentment and temper for half an hour after feeling put out by a disappointment and be "all smiles" after someone has made amends, the cyclothymic individual may feel low and appear socially withdrawn for weeks. A comparison of the frequency of mood changes is shown in Figure 1.

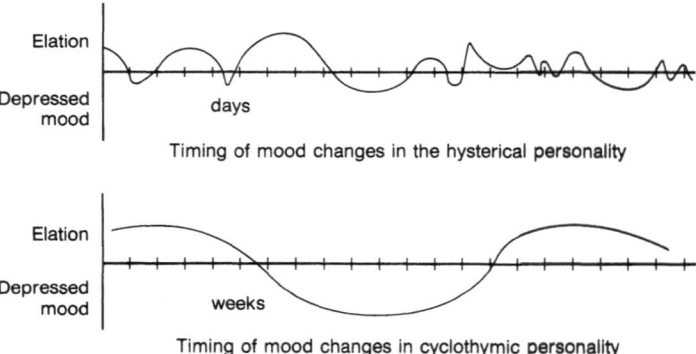

Timing of mood changes in the hysterical personality

Timing of mood changes in cyclothymic personality

Figure 1

Consequently it is best to think of the cyclothymic person as suffering from a cyclical alteration of mood setting rather than an unstable and easily alterable mood level. The cyclothymic remains stable in low or high mood, but may switch, over a day or so, to the other level without apparent reason.

The complaint is likely to be of the low phases which interfere with work, relationships and progress in general, much to the dismay of close relatives.

B. **MOODINESS AS A NEW DEVELOPMENT**

Psychiatric illnesses

i. Depressive illness

It is always surprising to find the enormously wide variety of mood changes which can occur in depressive illnesses. Not only do they span the range from violence to stupor, but there are subtle intermediate changes such as negativistic repartee, uncalled-for bitterness and vengeful leanings. A further complexity to this area is the frequent occurrence of panic attacks, pathological anxiety and obsessions as presenting features in young people, features which by their dominance mask the distinctive features of depression. This very common illness, atypical depression, can underlie a large proportion of expressions of moodiness.

In these cases the real "cause" is rarely cited by the patient and a host of false situational links are expressed. Not uncommonly marital problems arise from the change in demeanour of one partner who projects the problem onto the other, thereby widening the gap in the relationship without foundation.

The moodiness in these cases arises mainly from a change in personality which depressive illness brings. The individual is "different" and this reflects especially on children when the mother is greatly affected. All types of "insecurity behaviour" can arise in these circumstances, all too easily attributed to school problems which lie not in the school but in the secondary, depressed state of the children.

The diagnosis is confirmed by the presence of persisting sleep disturbance, changes in appetite, weight and libido and a marked diurnal mood change, although it is usual to find about three of these changes in moderately severe cases.

ii. Mania

None can fail to recognise mania in full-blown form; minor but common examples of this condition **can be easily overlooked**. They often appear moody but do not complain directly.

Relatives, puzzled by the development of moodiness or unusual behaviour, complain, often much too late.

In subdued form the patient may just seem irresponsible, but the clue is that it is seen in people previously most responsible and concerned about good standards. One hears of staid middle-aged citizens suddenly being found in conversation with strangers, flirting with the opposite sex, talking loudly and aggressively and showing uncharacteristic intolerance.

There may be no delusions, but the person's attitude is one of superiority, condescension and domination. Needless to say, management is one of the most difficult tasks in medicine and psychiatry, because of the patient's sense of omniscience coupled with a total lack of insight into the change which has taken place in themselves.

These patients show a sudden change in demeanour when they are thwarted. The elated, hearty, noisy person full of joie de vivre and personal warmth can change suddenly into an aggressive, abusive and violent adversary turning his or her energy from undue familiarity to equally unjustified hostility.

Friends and close relatives are those most likely to try to keep these patients out of trouble and from making fools of themselves, and they are prime targets for attacks. When violence arises, it is as well to recall that these patients have "the strength of ten" and should only be approached with great caution and never unaccompanied.

iii. Schizophrenia

Moodiness is a striking feature of early schizophrenia, and because the illness usually starts in adolescence when moodiness is an accepted feature, the earliest stage of the illness can be overlooked or the behaviour rationalised. The patient may show sudden swings of mood from elation to depression with suicidal intent over a short time, these changes being part of "incongruity of affect" in which the mood does not fit the thought process (as perceived from the patient's talk).

Some patients appear moody and unsociable, retiring to their bedroom and losing touch with the family, failing to come for meals or to wash, and often showing purposeless repetitive behaviour, but others smile or laugh inappropriately or seem unduly angry.

These mood changes are attributable to the acute damaging process of schizophrenia and their detection is important so that treatment with phenothiazine compounds can be instituted readily. It is important to look for other features such as inappropriate emotional responses, delusions, hallucinations, feelings of unreality and depersonalisation rather than concentrate on hypothetical psychological problems. Otherwise the individual is likely to sustain personality damage and start off on the short pathway to loss of personal warmth to reach the emotionless stage requiring constant care.

Physical illness

i. Cerebral lesions and acute virus factors

The greatest catch in the whole subject of clinical psychiatry is the undetected cerebral lesion responsible for a psychiatric syndrome. Both acute and chronic conditions can cause difficulty, but whereas the acute condition soon declares itself in full form, the chronic slowly developing condition can remain hidden until special investigations are made.

Particular mention should be made of the common presentation of physical disorders in children as a change of mood. The child may become withdrawn, irritable, difficult or negativistic during the incubation period of a virus infection or (say) in the presence of enlarged infected tonsils.

It is essential to remember that mood change and irritability may also indicate changes in intracranial pressure whether from slow-growing lesions or acute developments such as meningitis, encephalitis or cerebral abcess. In adults, mood changes from intracranial lesions are usually more subtle and difficult to detect. A very slight change in a mature professional towards aggression at work from a slow-growing centrally-placed meningioma, or the facile, confused appearance of intoxication during a subarachnoid haemorrhage are uncommon but classical.

ii. Endocrine disorders

Endocrine disorders of all kinds are commonly associated with psychological changes, and mood is particularly affected. This may be explained by the effect of endocrine changes on the hypothalamus which is very closely associated with mood control.

There are no specific psychological changes which indicate endocrine disorder or the type of disorder, and the psychological effect of the disturbance does not bear a linear relationship to the severity of the endocrine disease. The vagueness of these associations makes it **easier to overlook underlying endocrine disorder** in patients complaining of depressive illness in cases of diagnosed myxoedema.

The common links are important. For acute changes, premenstrual syndrome has a pride of place and for chronic disturbance, myxoedema and the menopause are champions. Some women are sensitive to the effects of oral contraceptive compounds, despite the now lower incidence of such effects overall. The following endocrine disorders can be associated with mood changes, and in a small number these can be severe and of a psychotic quality.

> Premenstrual syndrome and (occasionally) midcycle or post-menstrual changes
> Hyperthyroidism
> Myxoedema
> Cushing's syndrome
> Addison's disease
> Parathyroid disease
> Hypoglycaemia

iii. Hormones

As the hypothalamus is closely associated with mood control and direction, and as it is responsible also for regulating hormone functions, it is not surprising that the use of hormones can affect mood.

Of particular note in this area are the effects of steroid hormones and oral contraceptive compounds. Corticosteroids are associated with both elevated and depressed mood which can outlast the period of administration. These mood swings can be masked and well beyond the degree which could be accounted for by the patient's improved condition or deterioration. Thus the use of a corticosteroid can be associated with a true depressive illness while fully correcting the condition which distressed the patient before.

Oral contraceptive compounds and mixtures vary in their tendency to cause mood change, and some women are much more vulnerable than average. Whereas some will develop a full-blown depressive illness which does not respond until the hormone is withdrawn, others show a shift in mood which is subtle but disadvantageous.

Psychological changes similar to those of the premenstrual syndrome are not uncommon and the trend is towards hostility, argumentativeness or paradoxical repartee which can seriously disrupt the very relationship for which the use of "the pill" was intended to promote. Management of the withdrawal can require much persuasion and explanation, for in a state of low morale the woman can feel that withdrawing "the pill" will cause considerable difficulties in the relationship and will be reluctant to worsen problems which she sees as causing the depression rather than being an effect of it.

iv. Drugs

In young people particularly, it is well to think of self-prescribed drugs as a cause of sudden mood changes. Dramatic changes can be expected from the use of LSD, cocaine or solvents.

Less acute are the effects of sedatives and heroin, but amphetamines can cause marked irritability and aggression once addiction has occurred and has a "rebound" effect on withdrawal.

Of the frequently prescribed drugs, tranylcypromine and imipramine can cause marked tension and restlessness. For this reason they should not be used preferably for already tense or agitated patients.

v. Life rhythms

Individual tolerance or vulnerability to disturbance of life rhythms varies widely. In every social circle there are those who seem to be able to "burn the candle at both ends" with impunity, and those for whom one really late night unsettles them for a day or two. During that time the usual mood is disturbed.

Certain rhythm changes, particularly when persisting over a period of time, are disturbing for all. These are unsatisfactory patterns of shift working, moonlighting and "jet lag", but excessive persistent dieting appears to affect vulnerable subjects similarly.

Index

229